Northwest Vista College
Learning Resource Center
3535 North Ellison Drive
San Antonio, Texas 78251

T5-AEQ-443

R
855.4
.W66

NORTHWEST VISTA COLLEGE

Medicine in the twentieth century and

34009001176982

The History of Medicine

Medicine in the Twentieth Century and Beyond

Alex Woolf

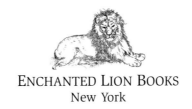

ENCHANTED LION BOOKS
New York

First American Edition published in 2006 by
Enchanted Lion Books
45 Main Street, Suite 519
Brooklyn, NY 11201

Copyright © Wayland 2006

Commissioning editor: Victoria Brooker
Editor: Laura Milne, Camilla Lloyd
Inside design: Peta Morey
Cover design: Rosamund Saunders
Consultant: Dr Robert Arnott, University of Birmingham Medical School

All rights reserved. Apart from any use permitted under UK copyright
law, this publication may only be reproduced, stored or transmitted,
in any form, or by any means with prior permission in writing of the
publishers or in the case of reprographic production in accordance
with the terms of licences issued by the Copyright Licensing Agency.

A CIP record is on file with the Library of Congress

ISBN:1-59270-040-3

Picture Acknowledgements. The author and publisher would like to thank the
following for allowing their pictures to be reproduced in this publication:
Getty Images: Taxi 3, Time & Life Pictures 5, 6, 7, News 9, AFP 11, Hulton Archive
14, Time & Life Pictures 16, Hulton Archive 17, Time & Life Pictures 22, AFP 24,
Hulton Archive, 26, 30, Stone 31, Hulton Archive, 32, Photographer's Choice 35,
Taxi 36, Getty Images 37, Hulton Archive 38, 42, The Image Bank 43, Hulton
Archive 44, Photonica 46, Reportage 49; Science Photo Library: S. Nagendra 4,
Peter Menzel 8, Philippe Psaila 10, Hank Morgan Cover, 12, Tek Image 13, Medical
School, University of Newcastle Upon Tyne/Simon Fraser 15, Saturn Stills 18, Andy
Crump/TDR/WHO 19, Zephyr 21, James King-Holmes 23, 25, Science Photo Library
27, St Mary's Hospital Medical School 28, Science Photo Library 29, BSIP
Laurent/Pioffet 33, Science Source 39, Dr P. Marazzi 41, John Cole 45, Andy Crump
TDR/WHO 48, NIBSC 50, Colin Cuthbert 51, Mark Thomas 52, John Cole 53, Mark
Thomas 54, AJ PHOTO/HOP AMERICAN 55, Chris Sattlberger 56, Mark de Fraeye 57,
Catherine Pouedras 58, Tek Image 59; Topfoto: Topfoto.co.uk 47; Wellcome Trust:
Wellcome Photo Library 20, Wellcome Library, London 34, 40.

*The website addresses (URLs) included in this
book were valid at the time of going to press.
However, because of the nature of the Internet,
it is possible that some addresses may have
changed, or sites may have changed or closed
down since publication. While the author and
publisher regret any inconvenience this may
cause the readers, no responsibility for any such
changes can be accepted by either the author or
the publisher.*

Contents

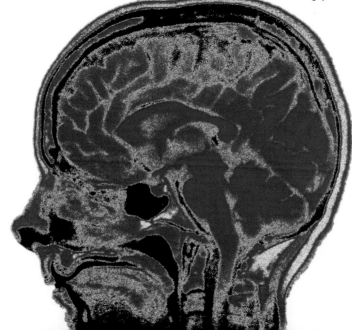

Chapter 1

The world of the twentieth century

A challenging time

The twentieth century was a time of great changes both in science and in society. Improvements in transportation and communications technology made the world "smaller." Scientists split the atom, harnessed radio waves, developed nuclear power and the microchip, and sent astronauts into space. At the same time, society became increasingly urban and cosmopolitan, with more people enjoying the benefits of wealth than ever before. On the other hand, world wars, genocide, famines and epidemics killed more people in the twentieth century than in any previous century. Also, the rapid pace of life, crime, pollution and terrorism made life more stressful.

Undeniably, however, the twentieth century witnessed significant improvements in physical health. Most people in 2000 were taller, heavier and better fed than their great-grandparents. Thanks to advances in medicine, the average person lived almost thirty years longer than his or her counterpart at the start of the century. So what were these medical advances, and how did they come about?

A nurse administers a polio vaccine to a baby in India. Polio, a major killer at the start of the twentieth century, had been all but eradicated by the century's end.

Medicine in the early 1900s

At the turn of the twentieth century, millions of people died each year from infectious diseases such as yellow fever, influenza and polio. Many more suffered from nutritional diseases such as beriberi, rickets and scurvy. Headaches and toothaches simply had to be endured.

In the early 1900s, a number of breakthroughs transformed this reality. Tests were developed for diagnosing infectious diseases such as tuberculosis. Chemical compounds were discovered that could treat these diseases. Meanwhile, scientists discovered the importance of vitamins in conquering nutritional disease. At the close of the nineteenth century, an effective pain relief was discovered by German chemist Felix Hoffmann. He persuaded the pharmaceutical company Bayer to market it, and Aspirin began to be prescribed in 1899.

Policemen in Seattle, WA, wear protective face masks during the influenza epidemic of 1918-1919. The virus killed 675,000 Americans—ten times as many as died in the First World War—lowering the average lifespan in the USA by 10 years.

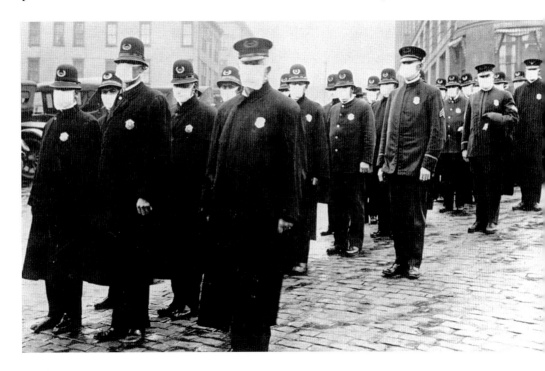

The influenza epidemic of 1918-1919

The most deadly epidemic of the twentieth century – and one of the worst of all time – began at the end of World War I. The influenza virus is thought to have originated in a military camp in Kansas. American soldiers probably brought it with them to Europe in April 1918. The powerful virus caused death within about two days of catching it. It quickly spread through Europe to almost every part of the inhabited world. By the time it ran its course in spring 1919, it had killed approximately 25 million people, including 12 1/2 million in India and more than a half million in the USA.

Medicine in the mid-1900s

In the 1930s, chemists discovered a series of chemical compounds called antibiotics that could kill the infectious organisms that cause disease. Penicillin, a well-known antibiotic, helped save the lives of countless wounded soldiers and civilians during World War II. The 1930s and '40s, were also notable for the development of vaccines against viral diseases such as yellow fever, influenza and polio. The discovery of insulin in 1921 proved life saving for sufferers of diabetes mellitus.

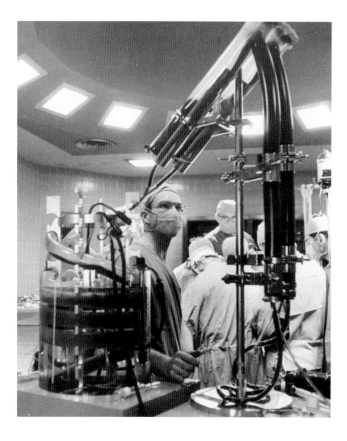

The heart-lung machine was invented by the American physician John Gibbon in 1953. This machine took over the function of the heart and lungs, opening the way to successful heart operations in the later part of the 20th century.

Thanks to improvements in drugs and medical technology, surgeons became more adventurous in the mid-twentieth century. The heart-lung machine made it possible to operate on the heart, while temporary artificial kidneys and an artificial heart kept patients alive during organ transplants.

Progress was slower in the treatment of mental illness. In the 1930s, psychiatrists began using controversial techniques such as lobotomy and electroconvulsive therapy, which are very rarely used today. It was only in the 1950s that drugs began to be developed for mental illnesses such as schizophrenia.

Medicine in the late-1900s

Potentially the most significant medical advance of the late twentieth century arose from the identification of DNA in 1953. This led to a clearer understanding of genes and how they effect heredity, which may yet lead to new ways to treat or prevent disease.

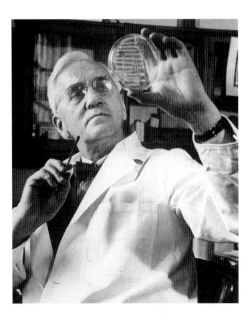

British scientist Alexander Fleming discovered penicillin in 1928. He tested it successfully on animals and even used it to cure a colleague's eye infection. However, he was unable to mass-produce the drug, and it did not come into widespread use until 1944.

New techniques allowed surgeons to use less invasive surgery, reducing the amount of anesthesia required and shortening recovery times. From the 1970s, methods such as ultrasound and CAT (computed axial tomography) scanning have given doctors much clearer, three-dimensional views of the body's interior, improving the diagnosis of illnesses. Engineers have created sophisticated artificial limbs, joints, and heart valves.

However, medicine also faced new challenges. Infectious diseases such as tuberculosis returned in different forms that were resistant to antibiotics. The HIV virus was discovered. HIV could lead to AIDS, which became a worldwide epidemic in 1981. Poor diet led to growing instances of heart disease and obesity.

Cancer

Cancer is a disease in which cells multiply at an uncontrollable rate, destroying healthy tissue. There are over a hundred different types of cancer and it is a major cause of sickness and death throughout the world. Throughout history doctors have sought to understand and treat cancer, but it was only in the 1850s that scientists understood that cancers are a disease of the cell. In the early twentieth century, researchers discovered that cancer could be caused by exposure to certain chemicals. By the late 1900s, it became clear that cancer develops through damage to certain types of genes.

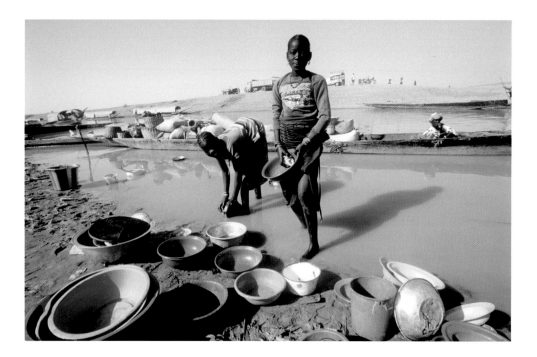

An expanding population

The twentieth century has witnessed a population explosion. In 1750, the estimated population of the world was around 800 million. By 1900 it was perhaps 1,700 million. By 1950 it had reached 2,500 million and in 2000 it passed 6 billion people. One major reason for this dramatic rise is increased life expectancy. Today the average person in the USA lives until 80, compared to around 50 in 1900. Some doctors claim that babies being born today will live to more than 100.

People are living longer mainly because of improvements in living standards. The world has vast inequalities, but more people in the developed world are richer than at any other time in history, and this has had significant effects on health. Human beings who are warm and well-fed are much better equipped to resist disease.

Wealth and health

If our wealthier lifestyle has had its health advantages, it also has created significant medical problems. If poor diet in the past caused sickness, today obesity—particularly

Two girls wash dishes in muddy river water. Many people in the developing world do not have access to clean water supplies and are consequently at risk from infectious diseases such as cholera and typhoid.

amongst children—is an increasing cause of premature death through its links to heart disease and diabetes. Excessive sunbathing can lead to skin cancer, and it has been known since the 1960s that smoking is a prime cause of cancer. Some research also suggests a link between mobile phone use and brain cancer—although this is not proven.

In addition, since the "sexual revolution" of the 1960s, sexually transmitted diseases (STDs) have become much more prevalent. STDs include venereal diseases such as gonorrhea and syphilis, as well as hepatitis, scabies and HIV/AIDS. In 1995 the World Health Organization (WHO—an international health organization) estimated that there are 356,000 new cases of STDs in the world every day, with adolescents most at risk.

Therefore, it might be argued that while improved living standards and better medicine have allowed us to rid ourselves of one set of diseases, we have replaced them with a different set of diseases and ailments through our modern lifestyle.

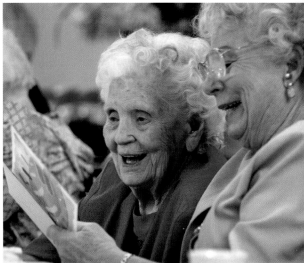

A Los Angeles woman celebrates her 105th birthday. The oldest person on record is Jeanne Calment, who lived 122 years (1875-1997). The American Census Bureau predicts that by 2100 there will be 5.3 million people over 100 years old living in the USA.

Treatments for AIDS

According to the WHO, 34.3 million people in the world have AIDS (24.5 million of them in Africa) and 13.2 million children have been orphaned by AIDS (12.1 million of them in Africa). However, there are inequalities in the treatment of this disease. While AIDS victims in the developed world are treated with a "cocktail" of antiretroviral drugs which can cost $15,000 a year per person, these are beyond the resources of African countries, which *together* spend only $165 million a year in total on all aspects of combatting AIDS.

Out of the forests

In recent times, mankind has encountered new and deadly diseases. These include hemorrhagic (bleeding) diseases caused by the Ebola and Marburg viruses, hantavirus pulmonary syndrome, Lyme disease and Lassa fever. In hemorrhagic diseases, the viruses destroy the blood cells, causing fever, headache, diarrhea, vomiting and massive internal bleeding, resulting in a very painful death. In the modern era of frequent international travel, these diseases can spread within days from city to city.

Many of these new diseases seem to be arising as human populations expand into previously uninhabited areas – particularly the tropical forests of Central Africa

Researchers collect the skull of a monkey to test for the Ebola virus. Scientists believe that an unknown host is responsible for human outbreaks of the disease. Certain species of monkeys, bats and rodents are suspected hosts.

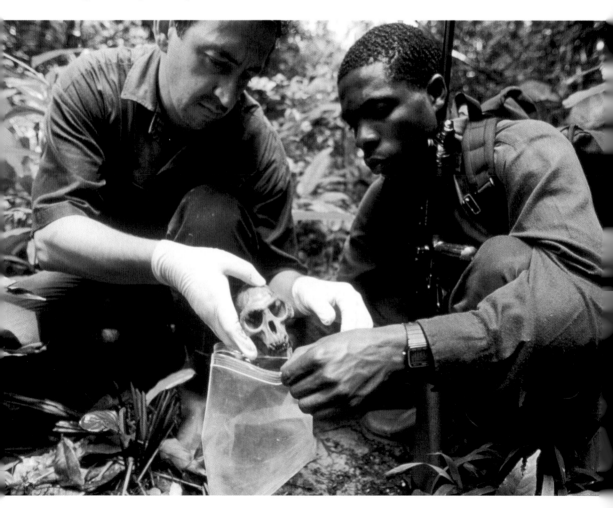

—bringing humans and animals into closer contact. The diseases have mutated in such a way as to allow them to cross species. Marburg fever, a hemorrhagic disease, may have come from green monkeys. Lassa Fever originates in rodents and is transmitted to human beings through contact with rodent faeces.

Other viruses seem to be learning how to infect human beings. Rift Valley fever is an influenza-type virus which before 1930 was restricted to animals. The human form of the disease, which originated in Africa, has recently spread into the Middle East. West Nile virus is spread by mosquitoes feeding on the blood of infected birds. From the 1970s, there were a number of outbreaks in Europe, and in 1999, West Nile virus appeared in New York City. Hantavirus, a hemorrhagic disease carried by rodents, has been spreading through the Americas since the 1980s. Avian influenza, a flu variant previously only known to infect birds, caused its first human death—a 3-year-old—in Hong Kong in May 1997, and by 2004 human cases were reported in at least 10 East Asian countries. Experts from around the world are watching the influenza situation in Asia very closely and are preparing for the possibility that the virus may begin to spread more easily and widely from person to person.

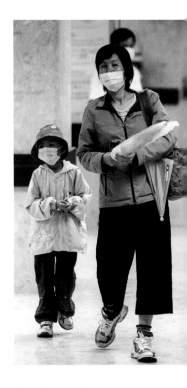

A mother and daughter wear masks to protect themselves from Severe Acute Respiratory Syndrome (SARS), a contagious disease that can lead to a fatal form of pneumonia. In 2003, a major outbreak of SARS infected 8,000 people in 32 countries, causing 800 deaths.

Donald Hopkins

American doctor Donald Hopkins (1941-) has devoted his career to finding cures for tropical diseases. During the 1960s he was part of the Smallpox Eradication Program, which helped to wipe out smallpox in 1978. Since the 1980s he has been in charge of the Carter Center's Guinea Worm Eradication Program. The guinea worm infection is a deadly tropical disease which in 1986 caused the deaths of 3.5 million people. By 2005, the eradication program had helped to reduce that figure to just 16,000 cases, and guinea worm infection may soon join smallpox as the second disease to be eliminated by medical science.

Chapter 2

How did knowledge about the body improve?

Looking inside the body

In 1895, the German physicist Wilhelm Röntgen discovered X-rays, and their use in medicine as a non-invasive way of finding out what is happening inside the body was immediately recognized. Within two years, the American physiologist Walter Cannon had found a way to make food radio-opaque by adding barium (the so-called "barium meal"), and had used X-rays to follow the passage of food through the intestines. In 1973, the British engineer Godfrey Hounsfield demonstrated the CAT (computerized axial tomography) scanner, which uses X-ray images from a number of angles to build up a three-dimensional image of the inside of the body.

Other ways of looking inside the body have also been developed. By feeding or injecting a radioactive substance into a patient, doctors can obtain a PET (positron emission tomography) image. Moreover,

A patient is about to undergo a CAT scan. CAT scans display a good contrast between the different tissues and organs of the body. They are typically used to locate tumors. They also are used by doctors to monitor brain activity.

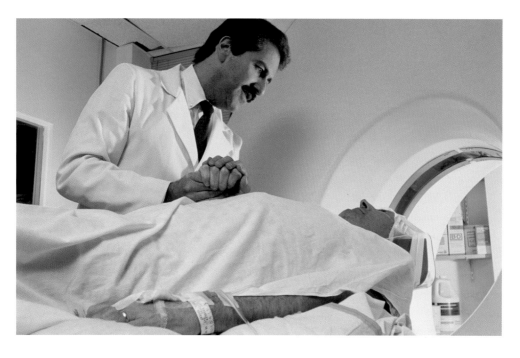

pregnant women can now proudly show their family and friends pictures of their unborn baby, as a result of an ultrasound scan.

Another major development has been the use of MRI (magnetic resonance imaging), in which a magnetic field constructs internal images of any section of the body at any angle required. These "maps" give doctors the information they require for early diagnosis of many diseases.

Blood Groups

The first known blood transfusion occurred in 1667 when the French doctor Jean-Baptiste Denis injected lamb's blood into three patients. In 1829, James Blundell, a London obstetrician, saved a woman in childbirth with a blood transfusion from another human. However, many patients inexplicably died, even when receiving blood from a close relative.

In 1901, the Austrian physiologist Karl Landsteiner discovered that there are different types of human blood, which he classified as A, B, AB and O. He realized that when the wrong type of blood is transfused into a human being, there is an immune response against it, leading to clotting, toxic poisoning and death. Landsteiner's discovery made safe blood transfusion possible for the first time. The first successful transfusions were carried out in 1907 by Dr. Reuben Ottenberg of Mount Sinai Hospital, New York.

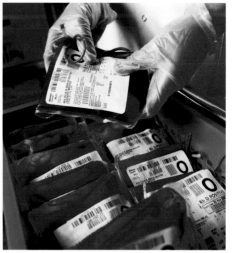

Bags of donated blood are stored ready for use. Donated blood is used in hospitals to replace blood loss, especially in treating bleeding disorders such as hemophilia.

Blood banks

A crucial discovery was made in 1913 by Richard Lewisohn, a surgeon at Mount Sinai Hospital. Lewisohn found that adding citrate to blood stopped it from coagulating (clotting), and this allowed the blood to be refrigerated for up to three weeks. This led to the establishment of "blood banks," places where donated blood is stored for use in transfusions. Blood banks have saved the lives of hemorrhaging patients, given help to leukemia sufferers, and enabled surgeons to perform longer and more complex operations.

Vitamins

Cures for diseases such as scurvy and beriberi were known about before the twentieth century. Limes had been added to sailors' rations since the 17th century to keep them from getting scurvy on long voyages, and the Dutch doctor Christiaan Eijkman, working in the Dutch colony of Java, had shown in 1897 that beriberi could be prevented by eating the husk and bran layers of rice.

But what caused these diseases? In 1901, the British biochemist Frederick Gowland Hopkins discovered the existence of what we now call the essential amino acids – organic molecules needed by the body but which the body cannot produce by itself. Five years later, Hopkins showed that rats did not grow when he fed them on artificial milk consisting solely of proteins, fats and carbohydrates. But when a small amount of cow's milk was added, they grew very well. Hopkins had proved that foods contained certain substances, which he called "accessory food factors," that were necessary for normal development. In 1912, the Polish physiologist Casimir Funk named these factors "vitamins," a shortening of "vital amines."

Developing Hopkins's work, medical researchers discovered a number of vitamins and the diseases linked to a deficiency in them. For example: vitamin C (scurvy), vitamin B-1 (beriberi), vitamin D (rickets), vitamin B-12 (pernicious anemia), vitamin K (lack of this inhibits blood clotting) and niacin (pellagra). In 1935, vitamin C

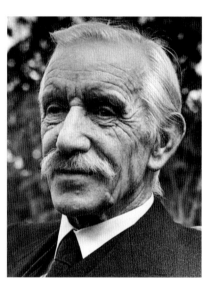

Sir Frederick Gowland Hopkins (1861-1947) was awarded the Nobel Prize in 1929 for his discovery of vitamins and his research into their properties.

Joseph Goldberger's work on pellagra

American doctor Joseph Goldberger (1874-1929) worked on cures for many diseases, including yellow fever, typhus and measles. He is best known for his work on the deficiency disease, pellagra. Goldberger discovered that pellagra is related to diet. It is caused by the deficiency of a certain nutrient found in such foods as milk, meat and yeast. He called the nutrient P-P (standing for pellagra preventive). Today it is known as niacin. He studied instances of the disease in isolated villages. He discovered that pellagra was more common in villages with diets based on corn – a poor source of niacin.

(also known as ascorbic acid) became the first vitamin to be mass-produced and made available to the public.

The discovery of and research into vitamins during the twentieth century has greatly improved diet and nutrition, leading to the virtual disappearance of deficiency diseases from the developed world.

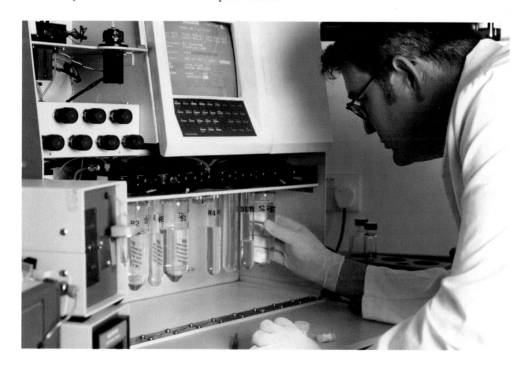

The Nervous System

In 1910, British physiologist Henry Dale isolated the chemical substance histamine. Histamine causes burning pains and convulsions, symptoms similar to those of surgical shock, and Dale discovered that it is released in the body by damaged tissues. Today there are a number of drugs that can suppress the body's histamine response, and some of these "antihistamines" are used to treat allergies.

Further understanding of the chemical responses of the nervous system led to the development of L-Dopa (synthetic dopamine), which is used to treat Parkinson's disease (a trembling of the limbs), and serotonin, which is used as an anti-depressant. Both these drugs work by mimicking key chemical responses in the brain.

A technician analyses the properties of a protein. Proteins are chemicals in food that the digestive system breaks down to allow the body to grow and repair itself. By studying the function of proteins, scientists can advance our understanding of nutrition.

Hormones

In 1900, Ernest Starling and William Bayliss became the first scientists to discover a hormone. Hormones are chemical substances that control many of the body's functions. Starling and Bayliss named the hormone secretin, which stimulates the stomach to produce digestive juices. Other hormones include adrenalin, which controls the discharge of sugars into the bloodstream, and thyroxine, an iodine-containing hormone that stimulates growth.

In 1923, anatomist Edgar Allan and biochemist Edward A. Doisy, investigating the development of the ovum, found that injections of fluid extracted from the ovaries could induce menstruation. They had discovered estrogen, a type of hormone that controls changes in the reproductive and sexual organs of females. Today, estrogen is the basis of the contraceptive pill and is used in the treatment known as HRT (hormone replacement therapy) to reduce the problems associated with menopause. Doses of estrogen can also help women get over strokes and slow the development of Alzheimer's disease in women.

In 1935, the Dutch pharmacologist Ernst Laqueur isolated the male sex hormone, testosterone. This hormone is used to treat male impotence. It also has been used (illegally) to increase the muscles and strength of athletes.

Wartime advances

A number of important medical advances occurred during the two world wars of the

Percy Julian's work on hormones

American chemist Percy Lavon Julian (1899-1975) was interested in discovering how natural compounds found in foodstuffs were converted into chemicals such as vitamins and hormones essential to life. In the course of his research he developed synthetic drugs that duplicate the effects of hormones, such as progesterone (a female hormone), testosterone and cortisone. Doctors use synthetic cortisone to treat arthritis and many other diseases. In 1935, Julian developed synthetic physostigmine, a compound found in the Calabar bean. Doctors use this drug to treat the eye disease glaucoma.

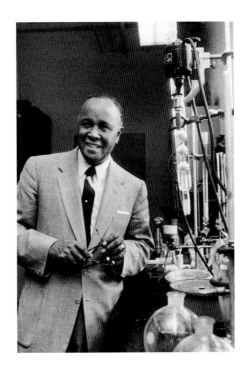

Percy Julian's work made it possible to produce drugs such as cortisone in large quantities, reducing the cost of treating arthritis and other ailments.

A team of surgeons from the American army medical corps perform an emergency operation in a dugout in the Solomon Islands in the South Pacific during World War II.

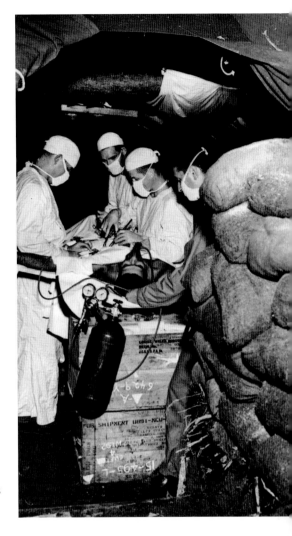

twentieth century. Remarkable progress in the field of surgery occurred during World War I. Large numbers of injured soldiers had to be treated in improvised operating theaters, testing the abilities of surgeons to their limits. They developed successful methods of draining wounds and cutting out dead tissue. A new wound antiseptic called Carrel-dakin Fluid was very effective in cases of gangrene. Advances also were made in the field of abdominal surgery, and successful skin graft and reconstructive techniques were pioneered. Perhaps most importantly, surgeons learned the importance of rehabilitation in the recovery process.

In World War II, a revolutionary advance in the treatment of wound infections came with the use of sulfonamides and, from 1944, penicillin. The war also saw the establishment of a blood transfusion service, giving surgeons access to blood in far greater quantities than had previously been available.

In the USA, World War II prompted massive government investment in medical research in support of the armed forces. Researchers made advances in a number of areas, including blood substitutes, anti-malarial drugs, and in the new field of nuclear medicine, where radioactive materials called radioisotopes are used to help diagnose and treat a wide variety of diseases. After the war, government-sponsored medical research continued in the USA under the National Institutes of Health (NIH). This program was further boosted by the post-war emigration of many talented doctors and scientists from Europe to the USA, establishing the USA as a leading center of medical research.

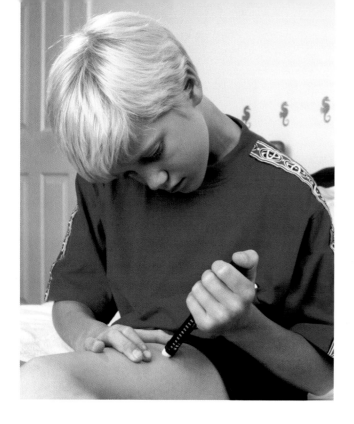

A teenage boy suffering from diabetes mellitus gives himself an insulin injection in the leg. Insulin helps convert blood sugar to energy. Diabetes is a condition in which the pancreas produces too little insulin.

Treatment for diabetes

Before the 1920s, diabetes was a terminal wasting disease. Unable to break down sugars in the bloodstream, patients lacked energy, urinated constantly, and were susceptible to strokes and blindness. The only treatment was to keep the patient on a starvation diet of cabbages.

Nineteenth century physiologists had noticed changes in the pancreas of diabetics, and in 1869 the German anatomist Paul Langerhans observed small patches of tissue in the pancreas known as the "islets of Langerhans." It was suggested that they were connected to diabetes, but nobody understood how.

In 1921, a Canadian physician, Frederick Banting, and one of his undergraduate students, Charles Best, discovered that the islets of Langerhans produced the hormone insulin, which was vital in breaking down sugars in the blood stream. With the help of biochemist James Collip, they learned how to extract pure insulin from the pancreas. Then, on 23 February 1922, they gave an extract of human insulin to Leonard Thompson, a 14-year-old boy who was dying (he weighed only 76 pounds). Leonard's blood-sugar levels dropped immediately and his energy and weight rapidly improved.

Immunology

Surgeons had attempted organ transplants in the nineteenth century, and skin grafts were common during World War II, but doctors were powerless if the patient's immune system caused the body to reject the foreign tissue. After the war, British zoologist Peter Medawar, then at the University of Birmingham, found evidence to support the idea of "acquired tolerance," meaning that the body learns how to resist a disease. He was to win the Nobel Prize for his work.

In the 1950s, immunologists built on Medawar's work to identify the complex mechanisms of the body's immune system. They discovered that tissues can be classified into groups in a similar way to blood, and that grafts and organs can be matched between donor and patient. In 1970, Roy Calne, a British transplant surgeon, discovered that 6-mercaptopurine (a cancer drug) suppressed the body's immune response. Other immunosuppressant drugs have since been discovered, allowing further progress in the field of organ transplantation.

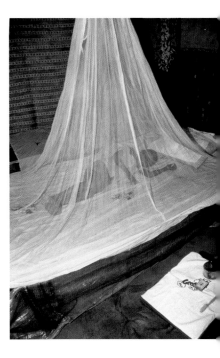

A boy sleeps under a net to protect him from malaria-carrying mosquitoes. Symptoms of malaria include severe fever and sometimes disorders of the liver, kidneys, blood, or brain that can prove fatal. Scientists estimate that between 300-500 million people a year are infected by malaria.

The fight against malaria

Malaria is one of the world's deadliest diseases, killing more than 3,000 people – mainly children – every day. Thus far it has resisted all attempts at eradication. In the 1950s and 60s, scientists used DDT to kill the mosquito that transmits malaria. They also developed drugs to kill the parasite that caused the disease. But both mosquito and parasite evolved to resist these attacks. Then, in 1972, Chinese scientists began studying herbs traditionally used against malaria. One of these – Qing Hau Su – appeared to work. The active ingredient, artemisinin, has turned out to be the most effective anti-malarial drug ever produced. However, because of Cold War rivalries and Chinese government secrecy, it took until the early 2000s for artemisinin to come into widespread use. Since the 1950s, scientists also have been trying to develop a vaccine for malaria. In 2004, they experimented with one that caused a 30% reduction in malaria cases – giving hope that one day an effective malaria vaccine may be possible.

Contraception

In the 1940s and 1950s, scientists gained a better understanding of the role of the sex hormones in human reproduction, and they used this to develop an effective method of birth control. American chemists Percy Julian and Carl Djerassi, working at the Mexican pharmaceutical company Syntex, developed norethisterone, a synthetic version of the female sex hormone progesterone, which was found to prevent ovulation. By 1959, researchers had created the oral contraceptive pill—a development which revolutionized not only medicine, but family planning and sexual behavior.

In the 1970s, the Canadian doctor Albert Yuzpe produced the misnamed "morning after pill" (in fact it can be taken anytime up to 72 hours after sex) which contains the active ingredient levonorgestrel, a synthetic version of progesterone. In the USA, this pill remains controversial and in most states it cannot be obtained without a doctor's prescription.

Contraceptive pills contain the hormones estrogen and progesterone, which prevent ovulation (the release of the egg during the menstrual cycle). They are about 95 percent effective at preventing pregnancy.

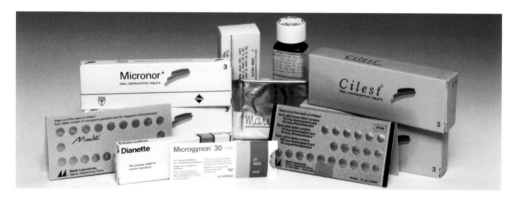

Reproduction

Biochemists also used the newly understood functions of sex hormones to produce fertility drugs, thereby helping infertile couples to have families.

In the 1970s, British gynecologist Patrick Steptoe learned how to remove an egg from a woman's ovary and fertilize it outside the womb in a process known as in vitro fertilization (IVF). The fertilized egg could then be replanted into the mother's womb. In July

1978, the first "test-tube baby"—Louise Brown—was born in Oldham, UK. She grew up to be a normal, healthy adult.

Women for whom pregnancy is impossible or health-threatening can have a baby with the help of a "surrogate mother." The baby may be conceived from the surrogate mother's egg and the sperm of the contractual father, or a couple can have an embryo, conceived using their own sperm and egg, implanted into the surrogate mother's uterus.

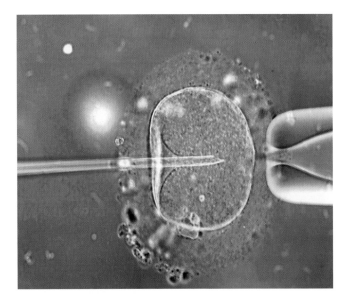

A sperm is injected into an egg to fertilize it in the process known as IVF. The fertilized egg is placed back inside the mother's uterus and the pregnancy proceeds as normal.

Ethical issues

Medicine's ability to make or prevent babies raises significant ethical issues. In the 1960s the women's movement viewed birth control as part of a woman's right to self-determination, and the pill is now routinely used, along with other contraceptive methods, even though the Catholic Church is against all forms of contraception. Should doctors be allowed to "play God" by granting infertile couples children? IVF is now an established technique, with thousands of test-tube babies born every year. However, many conservative and religious groups are opposed to it. IVF has given scientists the ability to conduct research on embryos in order to advance medical science and potentially find cures for a number of diseases—but do embryos have rights? A 1984 committee in the UK ruled that experimentation should be limited to fourteen days from fertilization. Many people still remain fiercely opposed to the idea.

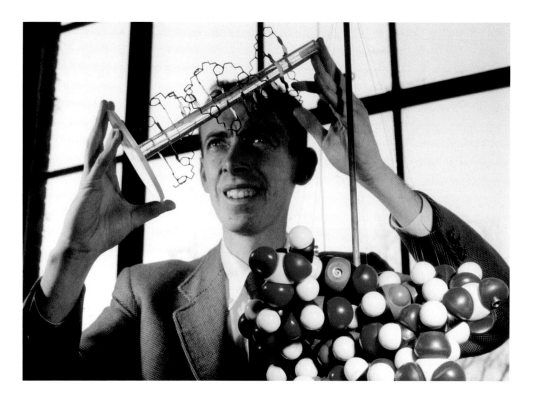

Genetics

Genetics – the study of genes and heredity – has its
foundations in the work of Gregor Mendel, a 19th-
century monk who showed how heredity is governed by
a set of basic laws. In 1909, the Danish botanist
Wilhelm Johannsen introduced the idea that organisms
had a "genotype," or a set of genes. Then, during World
War II, the American bacteriologist Oswald T. Avery
proved that deoxyribonucleic acid (DNA) is responsible
for the transmission of heritable characteristics, such as
hair color and eye color.

In the 1940s, American chemists Linus Pauling and
Robert Corey studied the structures of amino acids and
how they combine to form proteins. Pauling and Corey
suggested that proteins had helical (spiral) shapes. This
idea assisted Cambridge-based biochemists James
Watson and Francis Crick in their search for the
structure of the DNA molecule. Watson and Crick's
discovery in 1953 of the double helix shape of DNA
helped scientists to explain how organisms inherit

James Watson with the
molecular model of DNA that
he and Francis Crick discovered
in 1953. Revealing the double
helix structure was crucial to
their understanding of how
DNA copies itself into each
cell of the body.

characteristics from their parents. It also opened up new avenues in medical science (see pages 24-5).

In the 1990s, a number of "genome" projects were set up to map the genotypes of different organisms. Yeast was the first to be completed, in 1996.

The Human Genome Project

From 1988 until 1992, James Watson headed the US National Institute of Health's Human Genome Project – a project to identify all the genes in the nucleus of a human cell. The project also mapped the location of these genes on the 23 pairs of human chromosomes (the structures containing the genes in the cell's nucleus).

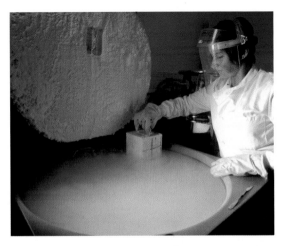

In 2003, the project completed the finished sequence with over 99% accuracy. Scientists discovered that the actual number of genes in the human genome is 20-25,000 – far lower than expected, and little more than twice the number found in the fruit fly. Moreover, most of the genes in the human body are exactly the same as genes found in animals and plants. As one scientist put it: "It comes as a shock to discover that you are 60% banana."

The mapping of the human genome may well revolutionize medicine by providing an understanding of the genetic causes of many human diseases. It is widely regarded as one of the greatest medical advances of recent times.

A technician working on the Human Genome Project removes a sample of human cells from frozen storage. The mapping of the human genome has given scientists a greater understanding of genetic diseases and should enable them to develop more effective drugs in the future.

Ethical and legal issues surrounding the Human Genome Project

The Human Genome Project has sparked an international debate on a range of issues. For example, does a company have the right to patent a human gene sequence for commercial use? Is it right to tell someone that they have a genetic defect that will eventually develop into a disease? Should an individual's genetic information be made known to insurance companies and employers?

Genetic engineering

Gene research promises to revolutionize medicine in the next century. By altering the genes of living things—known as genetic engineering—it ought to be possible to cure a whole range of diseases. This process has already started. For example, since 1982, human insulin for use by diabetics has been produced from a genetically engineered form of the bacteria Escherichia coli. Also, a genetically altered form of the cowpox virus has proved a safe and effective vaccine against hepatitis, influenza and herpes.

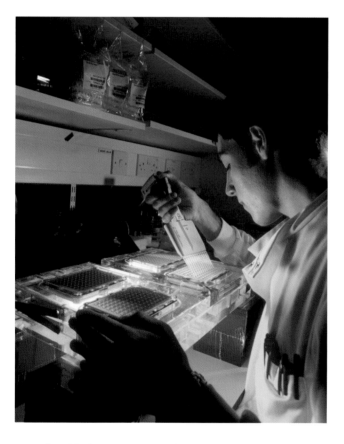

A researcher on the Human Genome Project. The medical benefits of this project are probably still some years away. Knowing which gene is responsible for a particular disease is no guarantee of finding a cure for it, but it certainly helps.

It should also prove possible to treat or prevent genetic diseases in the future by inserting genes into a patient's cells—a technique known as gene therapy. This prospect gives hope to sufferers of many genetic diseases, including muscular dystrophy, cystic fibrosis, hemophilia and some forms of cancer. However, there are dangers. In 2000, two children in France, who were successfully treated for an immune system disorder using gene therapy, later developed leukemia.

Gene therapy may also be used to treat non-genetic diseases. By inserting new or altered genes into cells, the cells can be instructed to carry out new functions. For example, cancer cells could be made non-cancerous, and immune system cells could be made resistant to HIV.

Stem cells

In the winter of 1953, Leroy Stevens, an American researcher investigating genetically inherited cancers, noticed a strange tumor on a mouse. The tumor was a teratoma—a cancer comprised of many different kinds of cells: skin, hair, fat, nerve tissue, even teeth. After further study of this and other teratomas, Stevens discovered what he called a "stem cell"—a cell that has the ability to develop into any of the different cell types that make up the tissues and organs of the body.

By 1981, researchers had isolated and grown mouse stem cells, and in 1998, scientists succeeded in extracting and growing stem cells from human embryos. Stem cells, with their ability to grow into any type of cell, might one day be used by doctors to repair damaged organs, grow the glands that secrete hormones, create disease-resistant cells in patients' blood, or even to grow into nerve tissue that would heal paralyzed limbs.

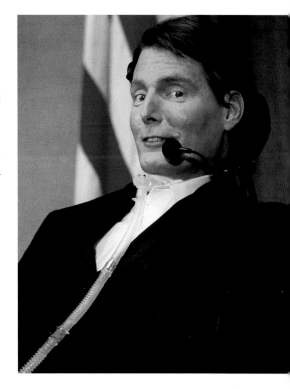

American actor Christopher Reeve (1952-2004) became paralyzed after damaging his spine in a riding accident in 1995. He became a campaigner for stem cell research, believing it could one day help people like him.

Engineered animals

Researchers are looking into the possibility of genetically engineering animals to provide new body parts for humans who need organ transplants. If a pig could be engineered to grow a human heart from the cells of the person needing the transplant, there would be less chance of the replacement heart being attacked by the patient's immune system.

Chapter 3

How did treatment improve?

Medicine by the 1930s

By the 1930s, there were significant improvements in the provision of health care across much of the developed world. Awareness of the importance of vitamins had led to better diets and a reduction in the incidence of deficiency diseases, and scientists were beginning to discover ways of treating infectious disease.

Yet these improvements were not felt everywhere. In poorer areas, such as city slums, diseases like measles, diphtheria, scarlet fever and tuberculosis were still rife, and doctors could do little about it. Many people continued to rely on traditional remedies, passed on by previous generations.

Chemotherapy

The challenge facing scientists in the early part of the twentieth century was to find drugs that were effective in killing bacteria but did not damage the patient. In

During the Great Depression of the 1930s, millions of homeless people lived in shanty towns on the outskirts of cities like New York. Diseases spread quickly in these crowded places, due to poor hygiene and sanitation.

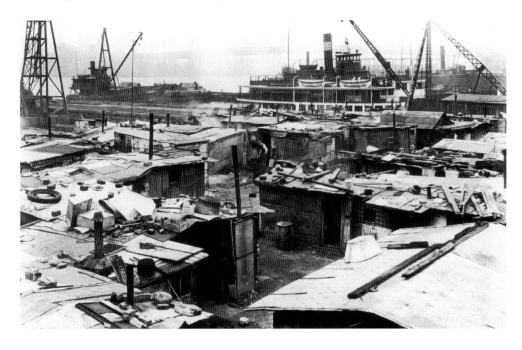

1910, German scientist Paul Ehrlich found that the chemical compound arsphenamine was highly effective against syphilis, without serious side effects. Arsphenamine, sold as Salvarsan, is lethal to the microorganism responsible for syphilis, and became the standard treatment for the disease until the introduction of penicillin in the 1940s. Ehrlich named this new method for treating diseases with chemical compounds "chemotherapy."

In 1932, the German scientist Gerhard Domagk was testing textile dyes when he discovered that Prontosil – a red dye derived from coal tar – cured mice infected with streptococci bacteria. Scientists at the Pasteur Institute in Paris found that the active ingredient in Prontosil was sulphonamide (a compound of sulphur), and that it worked, not by killing the germs, but by preventing them from multiplying, so that the body's natural immune system could kill the germs.

Other sulphonamide drugs followed, most famously M&B693, which saved Winston Churchill's life when he contracted pneumonia during World War II. In 1941, ten million Americans were prescribed sulphonamides. They cured not only streptococci, but also pneumonia, meningitis and gonorrhea. Sulphonamide drugs are still used today, notably in ointments for teenage acne.

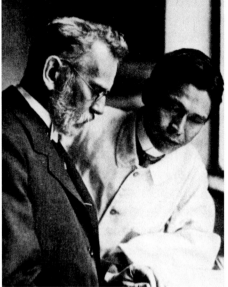

Paul Ehrlich (1845-1915), left, and Sahachiro Hata (1873-1938), the bacteriologists who developed the first cure for syphilis. Ehrlich had experimented with over 900 chemicals before he and Hata made their discovery.

The fight against bacteria

Ever since the French scientist Louis Pasteur discovered, in 1860, that bacteria cause infectious disease, doctors have speculated on how to kill them. In 1880, Pasteur discovered that *Bacillus anthracis*, cultivated at a temperature of 42 degrees centigrade, lost its potency after a few generations. Later it was found that animals injected with these weaker bacteria showed resistance to the more virulent bacilli. In 1885, the Italian doctor Arnaldo Cantani experimented with some success by painting one kind of bacteria on to the sore throat of a child with tuberculosis, in the hope that what he called "bacterial antagonism" would drive out the tuberculosis bacilli.

Alexander Fleming and the first antibiotic

During the 1920s, Scottish bacteriologist Alexander Fleming worked on the bacterium staphylococcus, the germ that causes boils, pneumonia and septicaemia. Returning to work from holiday one day in August 1928, Fleming began washing out some old Petri dishes when he noticed that a flake of mould that had fallen into a colony of staphylococci had in fact killed them. When he examined the mould, he found that it was *Penicillium*. From this he was able to extract the first antibiotic: penicillin.

Fleming's discovery is one of the most famous occasions of sheer chance leading to a great scientific

A photograph of Fleming's original Petri dish, containing the fungus *Penicillium*. The fungus's secretions, which killed the bacteria on the plate, became the first antibiotic.

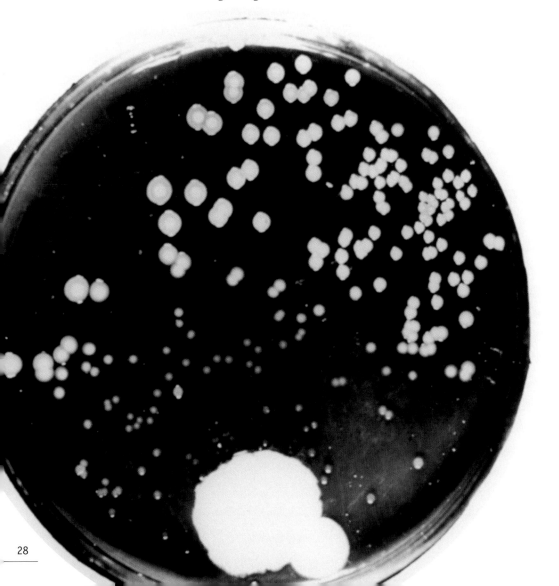

advance. Penicillin would have remained undiscovered if Fleming had not gone on holiday, if he had washed out the dishes before he went away, if it had not been summer, if the buildings in which he worked had not been old, or if the penicillin had not dropped into that particular dish.

Although he reported his findings, Fleming found penicillin hard to produce in sufficient quantities or in a sufficiently pure form to allow for its use on patients.

Florey and Chain

Ten years after Fleming's discovery, Howard Florey, an Australian scientist, and Ernst Chain, a biochemist who had fled from Nazi Germany, began trying to produce pure penicillin. While they succeeded in isolating a fairly pure form of it and were able to demonstrate its effectiveness, they needed to produce the drug in large quantities for it to be of practical value. Florey and Chain enlisted the help of Norman Heatley, a British biochemist who discovered how to grow the antibiotic in beer vats.

By 1944, penicillin was in regular use as a treatment for injured Allied soldiers. Blood-poisoning was virtually eradicated, and mortality from pneumonia fell from 30% to 6%. Penicillin was hailed as a "wonder drug." Other uses followed—penicillin mouthwashes, ointments—even toothpaste.

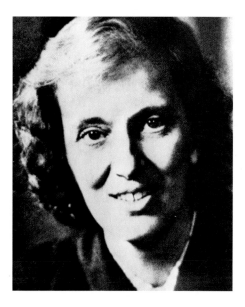

Dorothy Crowfoot Hodgkin (1910-94) developed a special X-ray method, which she used to determine the molecular structures of penicillin, vitamin B12 and insulin. She was awarded the Nobel Prize for chemistry in 1964.

Dorothy Hodgkin and penicillin

During the 1940s, British biochemist Dorothy Hodgkin discovered the molecular structure of penicillin. By doing so, she showed how the drug attacks bacteria and also prevents it from multiplying while having no effect on human tissues. At the time, chemists hoped that Hodgkin's discovery would make it possible to produce a synthetic form of the drug. However, it was only in the 1990s that chemists finally uncovered the complex series of steps by which penicillium mould makes penicillin, opening up the possibility of a synthetic form of penicillin.

Viruses

Viruses are so tiny that they cannot be seen by an ordinary light microscope, but rather require an electron microscope. They are about a millionth of an inch across, or one thousandth the size of a bacteria. While medicine's ability to defeat bacteria has grown, viruses remain generally beyond doctors' power. Exceptions include herpes simplex, the virus that causes cold sores, against which the first antiviral cream, idoxuridine, was developed in the 1950s. Another virus, herpes zoster (shingles) can be blocked by acyclovir, developed in the 1980s. Most viruses, however, including the common cold, are immune to antibiotics.

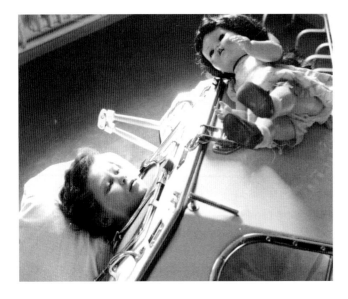

Polio can sometimes lead to paralysis as well as the inability to breathe. To help in such cases, American doctor Philip Drinker invented the iron lung. A patient would lie on his or her back inside a large cylinder and rhythmic changes of the air pressure inside the cylinder would force air in and out of the patient's lungs. Today, the iron lung has been replaced by a less cumbersome machine called a ventilator.

War on viruses

After 1901, the viruses that caused a number of diseases were discovered, including the viruses for chickenpox, mumps and measles, all responsible for the deaths of large numbers of children in the first half of the twentieth century. Doctors learned how viruses infiltrate the cells of the body, usually through the lungs, and then take over the cell's reproductive mechanisms to reproduce themselves instead.

Although no drug has been developed that works against viruses, doctors have managed to create vaccines that help the body to defend itself. By the 1940s, the electron microscope had been sufficiently refined to allow biologists to study viruses directly. The problem was that unlike bacteria viruses cannot survive outside a living cell, and so researchers were unable to grow them in a laboratory.

Then, in 1948, a team at Harvard University managed to get the polio virus to reproduce in the lab. This led American doctor Jonas Salk to develop, in 1954, the first vaccine against polio. After widespread testing, the vaccine was distributed throughout the USA, greatly reducing the disease. The vaccine proved so successful that by 1995 the Americas were declared polio-free. By October 2005, there were only 1,273 cases worldwide, and the World Health Organization hopes that the disease will be completely eradicated by 2008.

In the 1960s, American microbiologist Maurice Hilleman developed vaccines for the childhood diseases of measles, mumps and rubella. In 1971, he combined these into a single vaccine – MMR – providing immunity to all three diseases in one injection. Today, most children in the developed world receive the MMR. Hilleman is also responsible for many other vaccines, including chickenpox, bacterial meningitis and hepatitis B. He also worked out the pattern of genetic changes in the flu virus, helping scientists to give advance warning of flu pandemics.

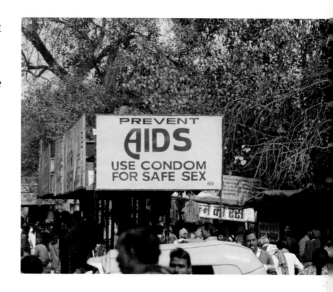

A sign promotes AIDS awarness in Delhi, India. AIDS is one of the most deadly epidemics in human history. By 2005, an estimated 40.3 million people around the world were living with HIV or AIDS. Between 1981 and 2005, more than 25 million people died of AIDS.

AIDS

AIDS (acquired immunodeficiency syndrome) is thought to be caused by the human immuno-deficiency virus (HIV). HIV is transmitted through bodily fluids, such as blood, semen or breast milk. The virus infects cells in the immune system. Over a period of months or years, HIV may destroy enough cells to cause the immune system to fail, at which point a person can contract life-threatening illnesses from infections that would not affect someone with a healthy immune system. The term AIDS describes this life-threatening stage of the disease. There is no cure for AIDS, but a number of drugs are available to suppress HIV's ability to reproduce itself, thereby preventing destruction of the immune system.

Sigmund Freud and psychoanalysis

The Viennese doctor Sigmund Freud (1856-1939) revolutionized our understanding of the mind. Using hypnosis on patients with neuroses Freud observed that they frequently improved after recollecting early experiences. Freud developed the technique of "free association"— talking freely about whatever comes to mind—to get to unconscious material. Freud also studied dreams and developed the idea of "transference," whereby a patient's feelings toward his or her therapist reveal feelings toward parents and other dominant figures from childhood. Psychoanalysis evolved from these ideas, which were expanded and adapted by many others.

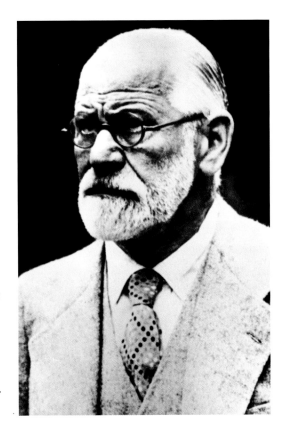

Psychoanalysis developed from Sigmund Freud's ideas and the notion that mental health problems can be remedied through talk therapy.

Psychosurgery

While psychotherapists made advances in the treatment of neuroses, patients with psychoses involving delusions and hallucinations, such as schizophrenia, were confined to mental hospitals, with few attempts made to cure them. This started to change in the 1930s, however, with the introduction of psychosurgery.

Lobotomies

The lobotomy was a surgical procedure developed in 1935 by Dr. Egaz Moniz to cure obsession and anxiety. It involved severing the nerves to the prefontal lobe of the brain from nerves in other areas. Moniz performed 20 lobotomies and noted that many of his patients became calmer. Then, in 1936, brain specialists Walter Freeman and James Watts took the technique to the USA, where the operation was hailed as a major breakthrough. Thousands of lobotomies were performed in the USA between 1939 and 1951. These were mostly on schizophrenic patients, although some were performed on criminals. Other patients included Rosemary Kennedy, the mildly retarded sister of John F. Kennedy, and the actress Frances Farmer. Freeman performed over 3,000 lobotomies, priding himself on the speed at which he worked.

The 1950s saw a decline in lobotomies as they were surpassed by new drugs. They also were rejected on humanitarian grounds, as side effects included personality changes, impairment of judgement, and a decrease in intellectual and creative ability.

Drugs

After 1945, drugs were used to treat mental disorders. The first effective psychosis drug was lithium, introduced in 1949 to treat mania. Several drugs were used to treat depression but the most popular was valium (1963). While drugs did alleviate symptoms, they were not a cure, proved addictive and had side effects (headaches and nausea).

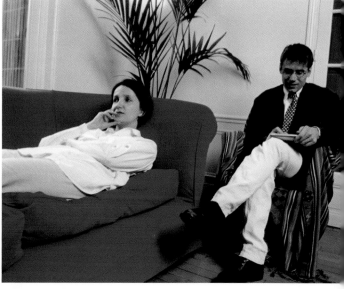

A psychoanalyst listens to his patient. Freud inspired many others to try to help people with mental disorders, and by 1980, there were more than 250 different kinds of psychotherapy being practiced.

Nevertheless, drugs have been effective in helping patients lead more normal lives, and because of them there has been a trend in the USA and the UK since the 1950s to release patients from mental hospitals allowing them to be cared for at home.

Behavior therapy

By the 1950s, a new type of treatment for mental illness had developed, called behavior therapy. This treatment is effective for people with phobias. It involves exposing the patient to a very mild form of their phobia and gradually progressing to the most feared object or situation. By the 1980s, behavior therapy was established all over the world, adding another useful technique to the array offered by psychotherapy and drugs.

Chapter 4

How did surgery improve?

Surgery in the early 1900s

The three challenges facing surgeons in the early 1900s were pain, infection and shock. Anesthetics such as nitrous oxide, ether and chloroform could be used to deal with pain, but many of these had unpleasant side effects. To combat infection, surgeons used a new approach, first developed in 1886, known as asepsis, involving the steam sterilization of instruments and materials. Rubber gloves and gauze masks were introduced in the 1890s. The third problem—shock— which usually occurred during a hemorrhage, when the circulatory system failed to supply enough blood to the various parts of the body, was a problem to which there seemed to be no answer.

A surgical operation around 1920. By this time surgeons benefited from asepsis, and the discovery of blood groups meant that patients could be given transfusions of their own type of blood to ensure survival during operations.

Surgery in the mid-1900s

Surgeons began to come to grips with the problem of shock in 1935, when they started transfusing blood during operations. Anesthetics improved in the 1930s with the introduction of the general anaesthetics cyclopropane and Pentothal, and the muscle paralyser, curare.

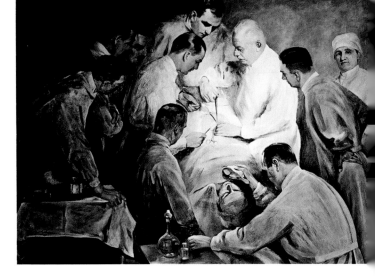

In the 1950s and 60s, surgeons built on the methods pioneered earlier in the century to perform some remarkable feats in heart surgery and organ transplantation. Operations on the heart had always been problematic because it was continuously in motion. Then, in 1953, American surgeon John Gibbon used a heart-lung machine to take over the function of the heart while he operated on it. The development of immunosuppressants (drugs to prevent organ rejection) made safe organ transplantation possible, and heart, liver and lung transplants were all performed in the 1960s, with a high rate of success.

Surgery in the late 1900s

Surgery in the late twentieth century was greatly helped by the implementation of monitoring devices during and after operations. These devices constantly check pulse, heart rate, blood pressure, and other factors to ensure that a patient's condition remains stable. Operating theaters today are kept fully aseptic, with all materials placed in an autoclave that subjects its contents to high-pressure steam.

New surgical technologies have been developed that supplement or replace surgeon and scalpel. Lasers often are used to destroy tumors and push detached retinas back into place. Cryosurgery uses extreme cold to destroy warts and skin lesions and to remove cataracts. Endoscopes, flexible tubes tipped with tiny cameras, can be inserted into bodily passages to provide interior views.

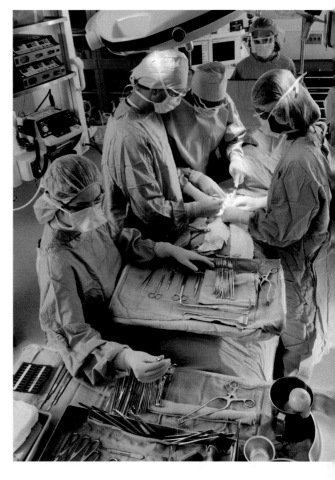

A modern operation. Today, surgery is far safer because the patient's condition can be constantly monitored during the operation. Developments such as CAT scans, endoscopes and microsurgery mean that there is far less need for risky invasive surgery.

Microsurgery

To operate on the smaller, more intricate parts of the body such as the inner ear, eye and small blood vessels, surgeons use a technique called microsurgery. In microsurgery, the surgeon observes the body part being operated on through a microscope. Microsurgery was first practiced on the inner ear in the 1920s, and the technique was advanced in the 1950s with operations on tiny blood vessels and nerve strands. In more recent times, microsurgery has been used to reattach severed limbs, repair the eye's retina and remove tumors in the brain and spinal cord.

Into the brain

Neurosurgery (surgery on the brain) is one of the most complex and difficult types of surgery. However, at the end of the 19th century, surgeons began to show that progress was possible in this field. By 1890, British surgeon Victor Horsley had recorded 44 successful operations on the brain. In 1893, Scottish surgeon William Macewen operated on 19 patients with brain abscesses, 18 of whom were cured—an astonishing rate of success at the time.

However, the greatest pioneer of neurosurgery was American surgeon Harvey Cushing, who developed many of the operating procedures still in use today. For example, Cushing carried out bloodless operations by using tiny silver clips at bleeding points as he operated.

In the 1950s and 1960s, brain surgery for conditions such as Parkinson's disease and epilepsy fell out of favor, as drugs became available

A magnetic resonance imaging (MRI) scan of the human brain in profile. MRI scans show thin-section images of the body from any angle or direction, and are mostly used to diagnose diseases of the brain and central nervous system.

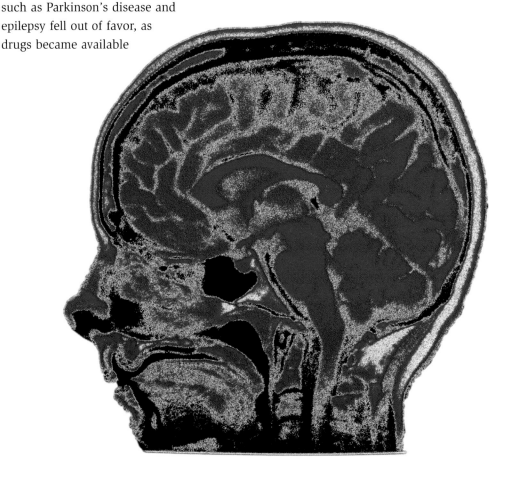

that treated these conditions more safely and effectively. However, since the 1980s, new brain-imaging techniques have improved surgical precision, and surgery has regained popularity, especially for those sufferers who do not respond to drug therapy. Today, surgeons use a technique called deep brain stimulation, inserting a probe deep inside the brain. A short burst of electricity sent through the probe normalizes electrical activity in that region, preventing the symptoms of Parkinson's disease.

Despite these advances, brain surgery remains risky, because so little is still understood about this highly complex organ. Many tumors, for example, are not operable, and even successfully removed tumors can leave patients with altered personalities.

Organ transplants

With improvements in skin graft technology, the establishment of blood banks and the development of immunosuppressants, successful organ transplantation became feasible. The first kidney transplant was performed in 1954, when Dr. John Murray transplanted a kidney from 23-year-old Ronald Herrick into his identical twin brother Richard. Richard survived and lived for eight years after his transplant. Since then, kidney transplants have saved 400,000 lives. 1963 saw the first lung transplant, and the first liver transplant, although both recipients died shortly afterwards. Today, more than 21 different organs and tissues can be successfully transplanted into patients, and every year over 20,000 transplant operations take place in the USA alone.

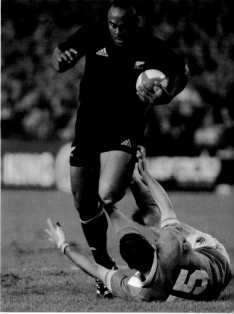

New Zealand rugby star Jonah Lomu suffered from a serious kidney disorder for 10 years before undergoing a kidney transplant in 2004. The kidney was donated by New Zealand radio presenter Grant Kereama.

Replacing kidneys

The kidney was always likely to be the first organ chosen for an attempted transplant. The fact that people have two kidneys but can survive with just one meant that donors were easier to find. And the invention of the dialysis machine in the Netherlands in 1943 ensured that patients could survive even if the operation failed.

Into the heart

Despite all the advances in surgery, many surgeons believed that the heart was a no-go area. As soon as the chest cavity was opened, the lungs collapsed, the heart went into shock and the patient died. In 1896, the British doctor Stephen Paget said, "no new discovery can overcome the natural difficulties that attend a wound of the heart."

There was gradual advance, however. In 1902, American surgeon L. L. Hill performed the first successful heart surgery, sewing up a stab wound of an 8-year-old boy. In 1929, a German medical student, Werner Forssmann, slid a catheter up a vein into his own heart under X-ray— a discovery which allowed endarterectomy (scouring the lining of arteries) and angioplasty (stretching a constricted artery). Surgeons learned how to repair the outside of the heart and, in 1948, the Boston surgeon Dwight Harken managed to push his finger into a heart to widen the valve between the two chambers of the heart.

However, the greatest advance occurred in 1953 when American doctor John Gibbon invented the heart-lung machine, which could take over the function of the heart, oxygenating and circulating the blood, during surgery. With the heart stopped during the operation,

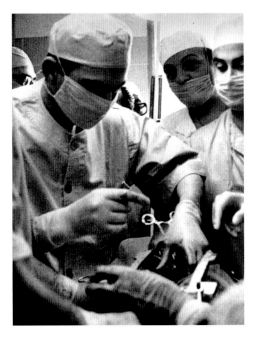

Christiaan Barnard (1922-2001) performed the first successful human heart transplant. His patient, Louis Washkansky, died 18 days later. He performed a second transplant in January 1968 on Philip Blaiberg, who lived for 563 days after the operation.

Mechanical hearts

Demand for heart transplants has outstripped supply, and for those patients awaiting donor hearts, surgeons have developed machines that can do the work of the heart, at least temporarily. Left ventricular assist devices help the heart to pump blood. Originally these were large machines but by the late twentieth century, they had become small enough to be implanted within the patient's heart. The next step for scientists is to build a successful artificial heart. In 1982, a patient named Barney Clark was kept alive for 112 days with an artificial heart. However, artificial hearts tend to make the blood clot, which, in turn, can block important blood vessels.

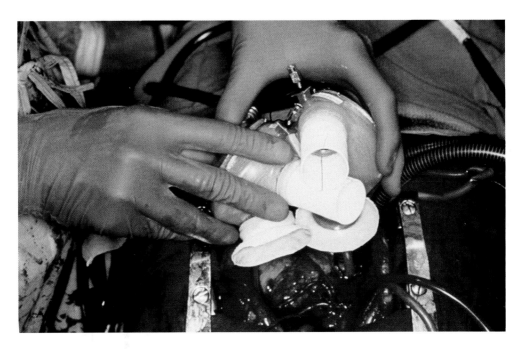

open heart surgery was possible. The heart-lung machine made many different kinds of operations possible, including valve replacement, correction of congenital defects and bypass surgery.

Heart transplants

Of all the organs in the human body that can be transplanted, the heart presented perhaps the greatest challenge to surgeons. A patient cannot survive more than a few minutes without a heart, and the heart is more sensitive than other organs to a lack of blood. The first successful heart transplant took place on December 3, 1967, in the Groote Schuur Hospital in Cape Town. South African surgeon Christiaan Barnard successfully transplanted the heart of Denise Darvall, a woman who had died in a road accident, into the body of 53-year-old grocer Louis Washkansky.

Barnard was ahead of his time. It was not until the immunosuppressant cyclosprine came into use in 1983 that heart transplants became widespread. Most patients can resume normal life six months after surgery and 84% survive the first year. In 2000, around 2,200 patients received heart transplants in the USA.

A mechanical heart, known as the Jarvik-7, is being implanted into a patient's chest. The heart is made of plastic and aluminium and relies on external power to keep working. The patient must, therefore, remain attached, via a lead, to support equipment.

Cosmetic surgery

The horrific injuries sustained by soldiers during World
War I encouraged early attempts at cosmetic surgery. In
1915, British surgeon Harold Gillies was the first to try
repairing cases of facial damage. Gillies developed a new
type of skin graft in which part of the skin is left
temporarily attached to the site from which the graft was
taken. This allowed the old blood supply to remain intact
while a new blood supply developed. In 1932, Gillies
took on his cousin Archibald McIndoe as an assistant.
During and after World War II, McIndoe treated hundreds
of young airmen who had suffered burns.

Now, at the beginning of the twenty-first century,
cosmetic surgery has become common and elective.
Many people choose to have their noses straightened,
their faces lifted and their tummies tucked. Breast
enhancements and reductions have become common.

Cosmetic surgery is now big business, and the people
who choose to undergo these operations are not always
doing so to correct abnormalities in their appearance.
Some wish to look like someone else. Others, wanting a
different look, ask for a nose job as a graduation or
birthday present: American teenagers alone had 42,513
such operations in 2003. In extreme cases, people have
even asked for animal features such as horns or a
forked tongue. This raises ethical questions. How far
should surgeons go? There also are physical dangers: in
1999 a judge awarded a $3.2 billion settlement to
170,000 women who sued the Dow Corning company
because their silicone breast implants had ruptured.

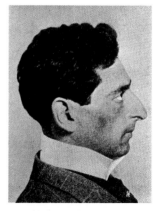

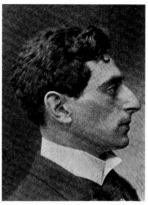

These "before and after"
photographs from a book
published in 1911 show an
early example of cosmetic
surgery on a patient's nose.

The Guinea Pig Club

Many of Archibald McIndoe's techniques during World War II were entirely experimental,
which is why his former patients called themselves the Guinea Pig Club. McIndoe cut and
shaped his patients' facial features freehand from skin taken from elsewhere on their
bodies. It was a heartbreaking time for many of the men. Immunosuppressants were
unknown, and rejection was frequent. McIndoe took care of the men's morale as well as
their surgery, encouraging them to go into town in nearby East Grinstead so that they
could learn to cope with the reactions of local people to their injuries.

Surgical advances

Surgery continued to advance throughout the twentieth century. Operations that once seemed miraculous are now commonplace. Cataracts once consigned old people to declining vision, but since the development of plastic lenses in the 1970s, cataract eye surgery has become completely safe and more than 95% successful. Since 1991, laser eye surgery has been able to correct eyesight permanently and do away with the need for glasses or contact lenses.

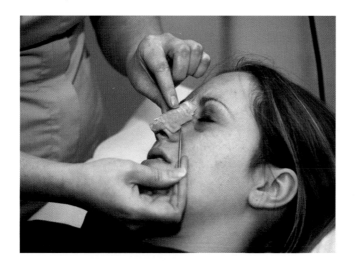

A nurse removes a bandage from a woman following a rhinoplasty. This operation reshapes the bone and cartilage in the nose to improve its appearance.

Surgeons have honed their skills, fixing broken bones with metal rods and plates, and even are able to mend bones severely shattered in road accidents. Severed limbs and digits can be reattached. The first prosthetic hip replacement took place in 1972. Today, 120,000 hip replacements are carried out every year in the USA.

Removal of the gall bladder is one of the most common operations. Today, laparoscopic surgery (keyhole surgery) makes this operation minimally invasive, dramatically reducing the recovery period.

Even more remarkably, surgeons now regularly perform surgery on unborn babies inside the womb. In 2002, British surgeons performed heart surgery on two fetuses several weeks before they were born, by inserting and inflating tiny balloons to open up sticky pulmonary valves.

Chapter 5

How did public health develop?

Health for the masses

Toward the end of the nineteenth century, as scientists learned more about bacteria and the causes of infectious diseases, efforts were made in various countries to control these diseases in order to protect and improve the health of the community. Major cities in Europe and North America established laboratories to study bacteria and develop immunization programs. In the first decades of the twentieth century, city authorities attempted to improve sanitation, reduce dangerous working practices, prevent diseases such as tuberculosis and improve children's health. This was the beginning of a modern system of public health.

In this 1930s cartoon, President Franklin Roosevelt is portrayed as a doctor trying to cure a country weakened by the Great Depression, and Congress is shown as a nurse. The idea of the government acting as a caretaker and nursemaid to the people was very controversial, due to the deep-seated mistrust of big government.

Community health services

Following World War I, countries such as Britain, Germany, Austria and Poland set up community health services, particularly for mothers, babies and schoolchildren. Public health nurses made regular visits to mothers with young children. The British government set up a system of "panel doctors" offering free health care to workers who paid national insurance. Similar national health insurance schemes were set up in other European countries. In the USA, where there was little support for a state health service, private insurance companies offered health plans and the government passed the Sheppard-Towner Act, which provided public funds for mother-and-baby care.

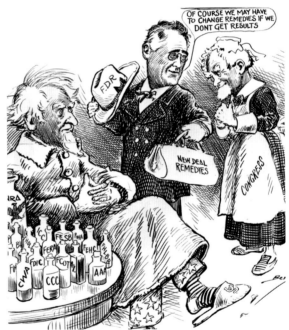

State medicine in the 1930s

In the early 1930s, when the Great Depression started to bite, some Western governments reacted by cutting public health expenditure. In 1931, the British government cut social benefits and reduced the fees it paid to panel doctors. In the USA, the government repealed the Sheppard-Towner Act. In 1932, a committee of concerned doctors reported that escalating costs meant that even middle class families could no longer afford hospital care, and that medicine was effectively beyond the reach of the working classes and many ethnic minorities. Yet the medical establishment remained opposed to the notion of a state health service. The American Medical Association dismissed the idea as "Un-American, unsafe, uneconomic, unscientific, unfair and unscrupulous."

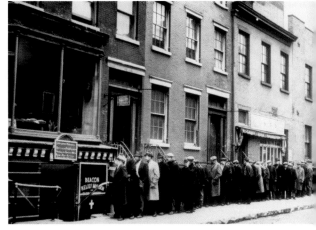

A breadline on a city street during the 1930s. The Great Depression caused serious public health problems, especially malnutrition. The health department in New York City recorded that one in five children were not getting enough food. Some even starved to death.

Nevertheless, as the Great Depression continued through the 1930s, and large numbers of people grew poorer, governments were forced to expand public health. In Britain, the government's response to the obvious hardships of the poor was to increase the provision of free school meals, provide free school milk and improve public health services. In the USA, as part of President Roosevelt's New Deal, the Federal Emergency Relief Administration set up rural health programs, and the Works Progress Administration (WPA) provided health care plans for its workers.

Public health in the Soviet Union

In the 1920s, the communist government of the newly formed Soviet Union set up an entirely state-funded public health service for the whole population. Each of the six constituent republics established a Commissariat for Health. Regular health checks were made on pregnant women, infants and workers in dangerous occupations. Large numbers of hospitals, sanatoriums and health resorts were built.

Britain—the National Health Service

The Labor government that came to power in 1945 was committed to the establishment of a welfare state in Britain. Under a welfare state, the government plays a major role in providing for the social and economic welfare of its citizens. One of the cornerstones of the new welfare state was the National Health Service (NHS). Established in 1948, the NHS provided free, comprehensive health care for every British citizen, regardless of taxable income.

Many doctors feared that the NHS would place restrictions on their professional lives. Nevertheless, most of them joined the service, and generally found that they had significant influence within it. The first twenty years of the NHS were fairly chaotic. It suffered from under funding and poor organization (it was split into 14 regional authorities that did not communicate very well), leading to inadequate patient care. Coordination between the regional authorities improved in the 1970s, but funding continued to be a problem.

In the 1980s, the rising costs and perceived inefficiency of the NHS became the focus of fierce public debate. Gradually, fees were introduced for items such as prescriptions, dentures and eyeglasses, undermining the founders' vision of a free health service. Over the following decade, the Conservative

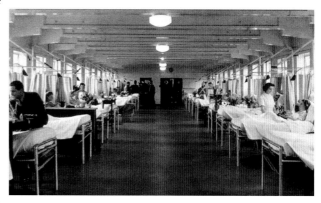

A ward in a temporary building at Guy's Hospital in London in 1948 at the birth of the National Health Service. This was a difficult time in Britain, with food still rationed and many buildings—including hospitals—damaged by bombs from the recent war.

How does Britain compare?

The NHS may have its problems, but it remains inexpensive by international standards. For example, in 2002 the UK spent about half as much as the USA as a percentage of its gross domestic product (total value of all goods produced within a country in a year) on the health service. Despite this, health in the UK, as measured by infant mortality and life expectancy, matches that in other countries in the developed world.

government tried to tackle inefficiency by introducing an "internal market." They turned hospitals into trusts and gave them the power to decide how to spend government funds. Under a scheme called GP fundholding, many GPs were given budgets to buy health care from hospital trusts. GP fundholders tended to obtain treatment quicker than non-fundholders, leading to accusations that the NHS had become a "two-tier" service.

In 1998, the Labor government began a new series of reforms. The NHS was given targets for expanding the numbers of hospitals, doctors and nurses, and for reducing hospital waiting lists. There were also changes to the structure of the NHS. Locally based organizations called Primary Care Trusts were given the power to run NHS services in their area. To pay for these changes, the government pledged substantial increases in spending on the NHS.

A modern NHS hospital in Chichester, West Sussex. Today's NHS has benefited from large injections of government funding, increasing the numbers of doctors and nurses and reducing hospital waiting times. Patients are given more choice over where and when they are treated. Cleanliness, however, remains an issue, and many hospitals have become breeding grounds for diseases such as MRSA.

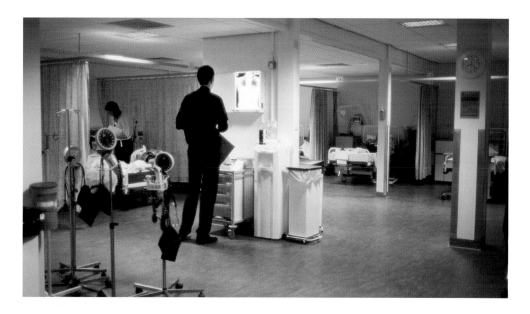

Today, the NHS is the largest organization in Europe, employing about 1.2 million staff, and with an annual budget of around $120 million (2003/4 figures). It is the most comprehensive, state-controlled, state-funded health care service in the Western world, with only 5% of NHS revenue coming from charges.

America—private provision

Unlike Britain, in America there has always been significant opposition from the medical profession to a state health care system. Instead, most Americans take out private insurance to fund their medical needs. For most of the twentieth century there was no federal health care provision for those Americans who could not afford private health insurance.

Opposition from the medical establishment prevented a national health insurance plan from being included within the 1935 Social Security Act. Similar pressure kept such a program from being introduced during the 1940s and 50s. Despite this, the federal government did begin to play a greater role in providing health care. In 1946, under the Hill-Burton Act, the government provided funds to modernize hospitals. Since 1946, it has provided more than $7 billion in grants and loans, which has paid for nearly 6,800 health care facilities in over 4,000 communities.

In the 1950s, public support for national health insurance increased, and in 1960 the Kerr-Mills Act was passed providing federal support for state medical programs aimed at the elderly poor. During the early 1960s, there was a growing consensus that a federal health insurance program was necessary.

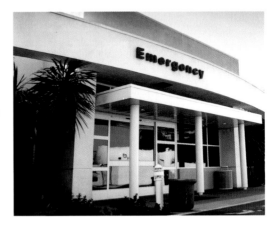

The emergency department of an American hospital. In the United States, hospitals and other medical services are funded by public funds and private insurance companies, as well as by individual gifts and foundations.

Falling through the net

Millions of Americans cannot afford private health insurance, and yet do not qualify for Medicare or Medicaid. Each year some 200,000 people are turned away from hospital emergency rooms as a result. Half a million American mothers give birth every year without medical insurance, and so are not covered if something goes wrong, and 11 million children are not covered by medical insurance. Yet when President Clinton tried to extend Medicaid in 1992-1994, he failed. The costs were simply too high for Congress to accept.

Medicare and Medicaid

In the mid-1960s, two programs were introduced—Medicare, providing health care for those over 65, and Medicaid, providing health care for the poor. Medicare is funded partly by taxes and partly by payments from those who use the service. In 1973, it was extended to people under 65 with certain kinds of disabilities. Medicaid is almost entirely publicly funded. It is administered by state health agencies, and each state decides what services it will offer.

Today, more than 80 million Americans benefit from Medicare and Medicaid. However, both programs have been criticized for inefficiency and spiralling costs. In an attempt to increase its efficiency, Medicare was opened up to competition from private health insurers in 2003. And for the first time, wealthier recipients of Medicare were required to pay more for services. Attempts also have been made at state level to limit eligibility for Medicaid and restrict the services offered. Since 2003, Medicaid recipients have been expected to pay reduced prices for prescription drugs.

In the USA, vast sums are spent on health care. In 2002, health care expenditure amounted to 14.6% of the gross domestic product—higher than any other country in the world—and some 4.5 million Americans worked in health care services. However, in the same year, only 41% of medical spending in the USA came from federal funds, compared to 83.4% in the UK.

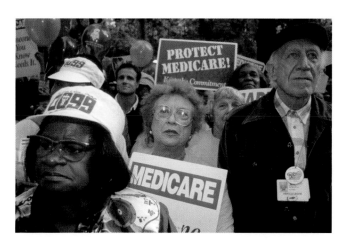

A demonstration against proposed cuts in Medicare in 1995. Since the 1980s, government attempts to reduce the costs of this program have met with stubborn resistance.

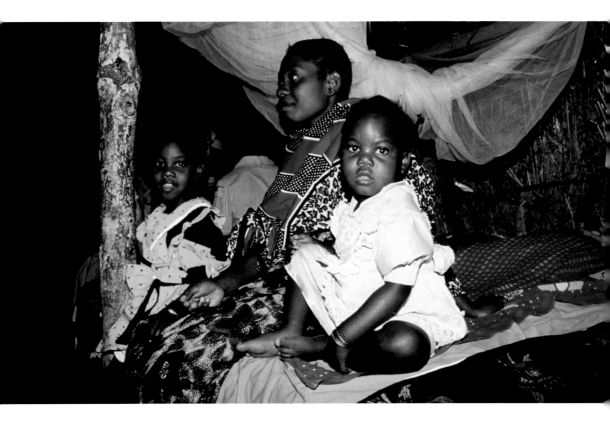

Health care systems around the world

Most developed nations established a system of public health care during the twentieth century, administered by the state and paid for by compulsory national health insurance (NHI). In some cases, funding is a combination of NHI and private health insurance. In New Zealand, for example, NHI covers most hospital treatment in full, but only pays for part of the cost of GPs and specialist hospital treatment.

Canada's system of NHI was created between 1968 and 1971. Each province has its own system – some voluntary, some compulsory. Almost all Canadians are covered for major medical expenses, with additional private health insurance for those who can afford it.

Australia's NHI system, called Medicare, was introduced in 1984. It covers the costs of basic hospital and health care. Private health insurance is needed to pay for services such as private hospital treatment, dental work and eyeglasses.

A young patient (right) recovers from malaria in a village hospital in Tanzania. The emergence of drug-resistant strains of the malaria parasite have caused a resurgence of the disease, which kills around a million children in Africa every year.

World Health Organization

The World Health Organization (WHO) is an agency of the United Nations. Its job is to organize and provide funds for health care programs and medical research around the world, to work to reduce disease, improve nutrition and provide emergency aid during disasters.

The idea of an international health organization was put forward at a United Nations conference in 1945, and the WHO was formally set up in 1948. In the 1950s, it embarked on programs aimed at fighting global diseases such as smallpox, yellow fever, malaria, plague and cholera. It also expanded existing immunization programs for measles, tetanus, tuberculosis, polio, diphtheria and whooping cough.

In 1967, the WHO embarked on a campaign to eradicate smallpox, introducing mass immunization programs in many developing countries. By 1979, smallpox had been eradicated worldwide. In the 1980s, the WHO launched campaigns to eliminate polio and leprosy and to fight the spread of AIDS. In 1996, it set up a division to confront emerging diseases such as the Ebola and Marburg viruses. In 2003, it led the fight against the SARS outbreak in east Asia.

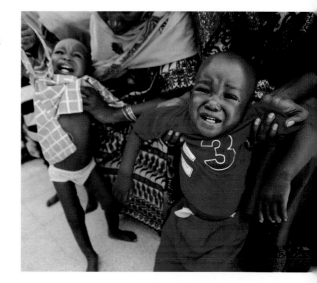

Children with polio await treatment at a hospital in Kano, Nigeria. Healthworkers had hoped to eradicate the disease by 2005, but it has reemerged in Kano where local Islamic leaders banned the polio vaccine in 2003.

Health care in India

The job of establishing a system of national health care is much more difficult in developing countries, which lack the resources for such programs. In India, the job is made harder by the size of the country, and by the sheer number and remoteness of its many rural communities. The Indian Ministry of Health coordinates a program in which thousands of these communities are supplied with "village health guides" and community health centers. In the absence of a National Health Service, this program depends on community involvement, charity donations and the service of voluntary workers. Deprived areas receive extra funds from the Ministry of Health.

Chapter 6

The twentieth century and beyond

How successful was medicine in the twentieth century?

During the twentieth century, massive strides were made in almost every area of medicine. Drugs have been developed that can kill infectious disease and contain and reduce the effects of mental illness. Improvements in our understanding of diet and nutrition have helped to rid the developed world of many deficiency diseases. Advances in surgical techniques and medical technology have enabled breakthroughs in the fields of organ transplantation and heart surgery. And our understanding of genes has opened up new avenues for the treatment or prevention of disease.

A team of researchers work on the development of potential anti-cancer drugs. Thanks in part to cancer research, 60 percent of people with cancer now survive for more than five years.

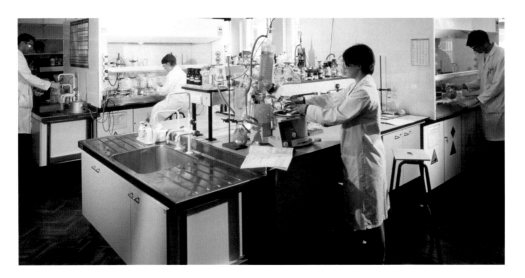

However, at the start of the twenty-first century, there are still major medical challenges to be overcome. Social changes in Western society have led to a substantial increase in sexually transmitted diseases such as gonorrhea, chlamydia and HIV/AIDS. The effects of HIV can be suppressed, but thus far the virus has resisted all attempts to kill it.

The wide availability of foods that are high in fat and sugar has caused a huge rise in the number of people suffering from obesity and obesity-related illnesses such as diabetes and heart disease.

Cancer

Cancer remains another formidable challenge. Since the start of the century, huge sums have been poured into research to find a cure for cancer. Public campaigns have tried to teach people about the dangers of smoking and to reduce consumption of carcinogens. Doctors have tried many different methods of treatment ranging from chemotherapy to lasers, microwaves and surgery. An exciting breakthrough has been the development of a vaccine to protect women from cervical cancer, the second most common cancer in women under 35 in the USA & the UK. Clinical trials of the vaccine are continuing, and if successful, the vaccine could be available within 5 years.

Yet despite this massive and continuing effort, on the whole little progress has been made. Although early detection has improved survival rates, only childhood leukemia and testicular cancer can be said to be curable. In 2005, there were 1,372,910 new cases of cancer diagnosed in the United States. In the same year, 570,280 people died of cancer; liver cancer had only a 8% five-year survival rate; prostate cancer only 4%.

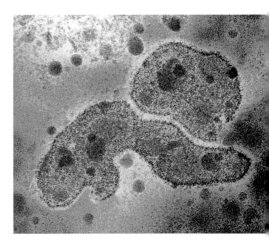

A highly magnified photo showing the H5N1 virus, responsible for Avian flu. Almost all infected birds die from the flu. Some humans have been infected through contact with birds, but so far there has been no known human to human transmission of the disease.

Avian flu

Avian influenza, or bird flu, is an infectious disease of wild and domestic birds. There are several types of avian flu, and in 1997, an outbreak of one type, known as H5N1, in Hong Kong, broke the species barrier and infected humans, killing six people. Other outbreaks of H5N1 followed in at least ten Asian countries, and by October 2005 it had infected more than 100 people and killed more than 60. There are great fears that H5N1 will spread to other areas, including Europe and America, causing a worldwide pandemic. A vaccine against H5N1 is being developed in the USA, but there are doubts whether sufficient quantities of it will be available if or when the bird flu strikes.

The practice of medicine

The development of modern medicine has significantly changed the role of the family doctor, or general practitioner (GP). At the beginning of the twentieth century, a GP was usually a man. He still made house calls, and still carried the tools of his trade in a bag. His job was to give the patient a correct diagnosis and to provide reassurance and considerate attention during the illness, since he usually could do little to cure the disease.

However, by the end of the century, 60% of new GPs were women. Many of the familiar diseases have either largely disappeared, or can be treated simply by prescribing a course of pills. All other kinds of treatment require technology, equipment and a scale of operation that can only be provided by specialist care. In America, by 1990, the number of GPs had shrunk dramatically: only one in eight active doctors was in general practice, and only 2% of all contact with doctors took place in the patient's home.

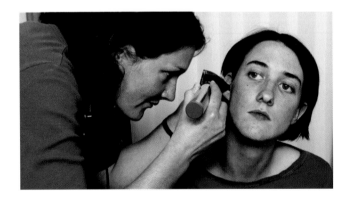

A GP examines one of her patients. The GP is the first medical professional most people will consult when they fall ill. GPs provide a wide range of personal medical care and refer patients to specialists when necessary.

GPs have survived better in Britain. In 2002, an NHS survey found that 82% of the British population had visited a GP at least once during the year, and that 90% of them were satisfied with the care they had received. It seems that medicine may not need doctors, but people do.

Hospital care

Hospitals changed a great deal over the twentieth century in terms of how they were controlled and run and the types of service they offered. Hospitals faced a financial crisis during the Great Depression of the 1930s, when many people could not afford the cost of hospital care. In the USA, the Blue Cross Plan – a form of prepayment insurance – was introduced in 1929 to help patients pay their hospital bills.

During World War II, hospitals suffered from overcrowding. In Britain, hospitals were reorganized by the Emergency Medical Service, and placed under more centralized control – a system which continued with the establishment of the NHS in 1948. In the USA, the Hill-Burton Act of 1946 provided for federal funds to help states pay for the building of new hospitals and the enlarging and modernizing of existing ones.

In the 1960s, as the role of the GP began to decline in the USA, many hospitals set up outpatient clinics offering general family care. Hospitals began providing laboratory tests, X-rays and therapy for outpatients. Since the 1970s, governments in the UK and USA have become concerned about the high cost and inefficiency of hospitals. In 1974, the US Senate revealed that 2.4 million unnecessary operations were performed in America each year, at a cost of nearly $4 billion. In the 1980s, the US government introduced a system in which hospitals are paid fixed rates for treating specific diseases. If the costs exceed the payment, the hospitals lose money. This has forced them to become more efficient.

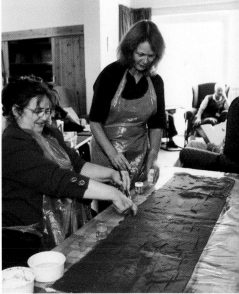

A patient taking part in a creative activities program at a hospice. Trained volunteers offer emotional, spiritual, and practical support to people with limited life expectancy.

The hospice movement

A hospice is a residential institution for the terminally ill, where the emphasis is on the patient's comfort rather than on curing them. Treatments offered include drugs for pain relief and spiritual counselling. The hospice movement developed gradually in Britain from its origins in 1905 with the founding of the St. James Hospice in London. The St. Christopher Hospice, also in London, was founded in 1967 by Dame Cicely Saunders. It became renowned for its tranquil environment and professional standards of care. Since then, the hospice movement has spread throughout Europe, North America and Australia.

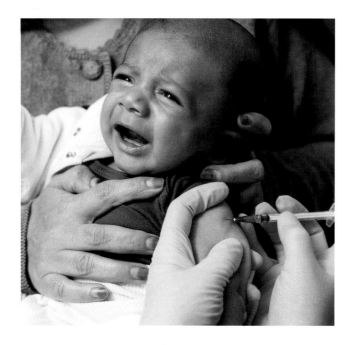

A baby is given a vaccination against tuberculosis (TB). The vaccine contains a weakened form of the bacteria that causes TB in humans, strengthening the immune system against the disease.

Drug developments of the twentieth century

From the development of chemotherapy in 1910, the twentieth century has witnessed spectacular advances in the treatment of illnesses with drugs. The sulphonamide drugs of the 1930s helped to cure such diseases as streptococci, pneumonia, meningitis and gonorrhoea.

In the 1940s, penicillin—the first antibiotic—was found to both kill bacteria and inhibit their growth, and was effective against a whole range of common diseases, including pneumonia, tetanus, syphilis, septicaemia, gangrene, gonorrhea and scarlet fever. Many other antibiotics have come into general use since the 1950s, greatly reducing fatalities from once deadly diseases such as tuberculosis and malaria. Antibiotic drugs have proved useful in treating cancer, although they often attack healthy cells as well as cancer cells, and a chemotherapeutic cure for cancer has yet to be found.

Chemotherapeutic treatments for viral diseases have been harder to find, although new drugs have been developed for treating shingles and chickenpox.

Since the 1940s, drugs have been used to treat mental disorders, helping mentally ill patients to live more comfortable and normal lives.

Side effects

Medical drugs are not without their dangers. Many patients have discovered that they can cause unpleasant side effects or allergic reactions, and they can lead to severe illness and even death if taken in too great a quantity. Occasionally drugs have been introduced that have unforeseen side effects. Perhaps the worst example was thalidomide, marketed in the 1950s as a "safe" sleeping tablet for pregnant women. By 1961, it was realized with horror that thalidomide was responsible for a sudden increase in phocomelia (literally "seal extremities") in babies born with limbs so shortened that their hands and feet seemed to be attached to the body.

There have been other examples. In 1971, US officials announced that the synthetic estrogen drug DES, given to pregnant women since the 1940s to prevent miscarriages, caused vaginal cancer in some women. By 1961, doctors had realized that the contraceptive pill could cause thromboses, phlebitis, migraine and jaundice. In 1997 the appetite suppressant Phen Fen (the so called "diet drug") had to be taken off the market because it was found to cause irreparable heart valve damage.

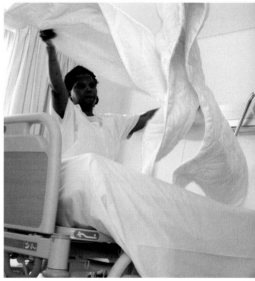

A cleaner changes the sheets on a hospital bed. Hospitals can be breeding grounds for drug-resistant bacteria such as MRSA. It is therefore vital that vacated rooms are cleaned with great care, to prevent any spread of infection to future patients.

MRSA

Bacterial genes are constantly mutating, helping them to become resistant to antibiotic drugs. One such bacteria, known as MRSA (methicillin-resistant Staphylococcus aureus), resistant to a range of antibiotics, was discovered in many British hospitals towards the end of the twentieth century. Infection rates soared, and by 2004, 5,000 people had died. Antibiotics are not completely powerless against MRSA, but require a much higher dose over a longer period. Doctors say MRSA can develop when people fail to finish a course of antibiotics. If the course is not completed, the most resistant strains of bacteria can still survive. In hospitals, many different strains of resistant bacteria are thrown together, making patients who are old and ill particularly vulnerable to MRSA. The British government has tried to improve hygiene standards in hospitals in an effort to combat the disease.

Alternative medicine

In the second half of the twentieth century, increasing numbers of people in Western countries became disillusioned with conventional medicine because of its side-effects and risks, and its inability to cure some common serious diseases. Many patients disliked the way conventional medicine treated the disease rather than the patient, killing the infection but not strengthening the body's own immune system, thus leaving patients vulnerable to future illnesses.

Instead, many people turned to alternative treatments such as acupuncture, naturopathy, homeopathy, aromatherapy and herbalism. Such methods use natural remedies to heal people, in preference to "invasive" treatments such as chemical drugs and surgery. Other kinds of treatment explore the mind's ability to effect, and possibly heal, the body. These include meditation, hypnosis, biofeedback and faith healing. By 1990, Americans were making 388 million visits to doctors, but 425 million visits to unconventional healers.

Initially, many conventional doctors regarded alternative medicine with scepticism, doubting its scientific validity and pointing out the dangers of relying on unqualified practitioners. However, in the latter part of the century, as popularity for these treatments grew, and as their practitioners became more professional, doctors began to find ways of combining the best practices of both alternative and conventional

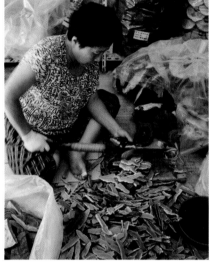

A South Korean herbalist prepares her remedies, obtaining extracts from plants and herbs to cure diseases. Herbalism, still widely practiced in South and East Asia, has gained limited acceptance by some Western doctors.

Healthy lifestyles

In the richer countries, ever more people are taking their health into their own hands. Gyms and fitness centers have become ever more popular, as have health farms and yoga practice. There is a trend among wealthier people for healthier diets, including organic and wholegrain foods, multi-vitamin tablets and decaffeinated coffee. Today, people are more likely to use medical facilities proactively, asking for screening tests, flu shots and health checks.

medicine. In 1992, the US National Institute of Health founded the Office of Alternative Medicine to investigate the benefits of non-conventional healing. By 1999, one in five Britons were seeking alternative medicine, half of them having been referred by their own doctor.

Global inequality

Despite the work of the WHO, and donations by Western governments of large amounts of medical aid, health conditions in many less developed parts of the world remain very poor. There continues to be a high death toll from deficiency diseases (easily cured by proper nutrition) that have all but disappeared from the developed world. Ten people die each minute from diarrhea, caused by polluted drinking water, even though the problem can be remedied by the consumption of a small pack of vital salts costing 25 cents.

The medical advances described in this book have really only effected the developed world. However, efforts are being made to address this inequality. For example, global funding to combat AIDS in the world's poorest countries has increased from $2 billion to $6 billion. The cost of anti-AIDS drugs has fallen from $10,000 per year to about $350 per year, making them more affordable for sufferers in poorer countries. By December 2004, some 700,000 people in developing countries had access to anti-AIDS drugs, a rise of 50% in six months. Yet nine out of ten people who need these medicines are still not receiving them.

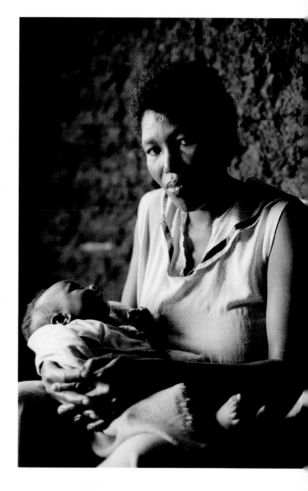

An HIV-infected mother with her child. Infected women risk passing on the disease to their babies during childbirth or breastfeeding. This risk can be reduced by the use of anti-retroviral drugs.

New challenges and debates

In the early twenty-first century, medicine faces a number of new challenges and ethical debates. The possible use of stem cells to help the body regrow nerves, arteries, tissue and muscles is very exciting, and may help future patients suffering from paralysis and even remedy the failing hearing and eyesight of old age. However, research into this area is most easily performed on embryos, and many people remain strongly opposed to this.

In gene therapy, healthy genes are introduced into a patient's body to replace unhealthy genes. In the future, this may be a cure for diseases such as cystic fibrosis. In germline gene therapy, healthy genes are introduced into a patient's reproductive cells to replace unhealthy genes there, and so prevent the patient from passing on an inherited disease to his or her children. This is controversial because it involves permanently altering the genetic code of both the patient and any of the patient's future offspring. So far germline gene therapy has only been tried on animals, and it remains illegal in many countries.

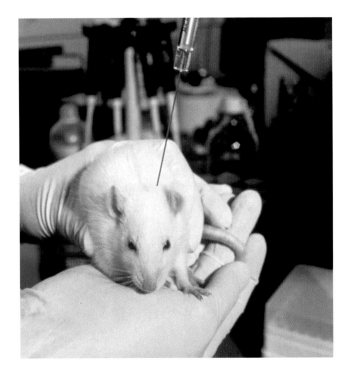

A laboratory rat is given an injection as part of gene therapy research into Alzheimer's disease. At present, the major drawback with gene therapy is that the healthy cells that are introduced into a patient's body only live for a short time, so the treatment must be repeated regularly.

In the future, as medicine advances, these ethical debates are likely to become ever more urgent. For example, our cells could be genetically engineered to prevent them from deteriorating, prolonging our lives. We also know that individual genes are responsible for characteristics like gender, eye and hair color, even intelligence, personality and ambition. It is likely that many parents, given the choice, will want to control such traits in order to have the "ideal" child. This kind of genetic engineering would probably only be available to the rich, leading to the emergence of an elite class of genetically enhanced, super-intelligent people.

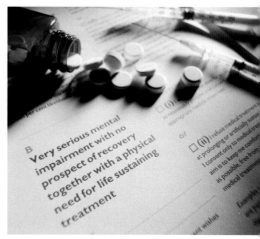

Medicine in the future

Over the next hundred years, medicine will advance still further in areas that we can only guess at. However, history teaches that the practice of medicine is as much a product of the attitudes of the day (such as religious beliefs and political convictions) as it is a reflection of scientific advancement. It can, therefore, be assumed that the development of future medicines and treatments will be shaped both by discoveries in the laboratory, as well as by the moral and ethical concerns of society.

A terminally ill patient who wishes to die usually needs the help of another person – often a doctor – to administer an overdose of drugs, either with pills or a syringe. Many believe that doctors should not assist in active euthanasia.

Euthanasia

Modern medicine has found ways of keeping people alive despite the most debilitating illnesses. This has sparked an increasingly fierce debate about the rights and wrongs of euthanasia, or mercy killing. There are two kinds of euthanasia, active and passive. Active euthanasia involves the painless ending of a patient's life for merciful reasons, for example when a doctor administers a lethal dose of medication. Passive euthanasia involves not doing something to prevent the death of a terminally ill patient. Most doctors now agree that patients have a right to passive euthanasia. However, active euthanasia is opposed by many, including religious groups and some lawyers and doctors, who argue it is inconsistent with the doctor's duty of preserving life and is open to abuse. Supporters say that relief from suffering, not preservation of life, should be the primary role of caretakers.

Glossary

Abscess a pus-filled cavity usually caused by bacterial infection

Acupuncture a Chinese method of treating illness by inserting needles into the skin at points where the flow of energy is thought to be blocked

AIDS a disease of the immune system thought to be caused by infection with the HIV virus

Alzheimer's disease a disorder of the brain that causes the progressive deterioration of functions such as memory

Anemia a blood disorder in which there are too few red blood cells, or the red blood cells are deficient in hemoglobin (an iron-containing protein)

Anesthesia the temporary reduction of sensitivity to pain in all parts of the body to allow surgery to take place

Antibiotic a chemical drug that is able to kill or inactivate bacteria in the body

Antiretroviral drugs a class of drugs that slow down the activity of retroviruses such as HIV

Antiseptic reducing or preventing infection by eliminating or reducing the growth of bacteria

Aromatherapy the use of oils extracted from plants to treat physical or psychological disorders, usually through massage or inhalation

Asepsis a condition in which no disease causing bacteria are present

Beriberi a disease of the nerves caused by a deficiency of the vitamin thiamine

CAT scanner a computerized axial tomography scanner that produces cross-sectional images of the body

Cataract a disease in which the lens of the eye becomes covered in a film that affects sight, eventually causing total blindness

Chemotherapy the use of chemical drugs to treat diseases

Cystic fibrosis a disease of the glands that causes the secretion of thick mucus that blocks internal passages and causes respiratory infections

Diabetes mellitus a disorder in which there is no control of blood sugar due to inadequate insulin production (Type 1) or reduced sensitivity to insulin (Type 2)

DNA deoxyribonucleic acid is a molecule in the form of a double helix that carries genetic information

Ebola virus a contagious virus transmitted through blood and body fluids that causes the linings of the body's organs to leak blood and fluids, usually resulting in death

Electron microscope a high-powered microscope that uses beams of electrons focused by an electron lens to create a magnified image

Embryo human offspring in the early stages of conception, up to the end of the eighth week

Epilepsy a disorder involving episodes of abnormal electrical discharge in the brain causing periodic loss of consciousness and convulsions

Gangrene decay of soft tissues in part of the body due to lack of blood in the area

Gene a section of DNA that gives a particular characteristic to a living thing

Genome a complete set of genes for a particular living thing

Gland an organ or a mass of cells that removes substances from the bloodstream and then passes them back into the blood in altered form for a particular purpose

Glaucoma an eye disorder marked by abnormally high pressure in the eyeball causing damage to the optic disc, which can lead to impaired vision and blindness

Gonorrhoea a sexually transmitted disease

Guinea worm infection a disease caused by a long thin worm found in Africa and Asia, that lives as a parasite under the skin of people and animals and can grow to several feet in length

Herbalism the use of medicinal herbs to treat medical disorders

Herpes a viral infection causing painful blisters and inflammation

HIV a retrovirus that destroys cells in the immune system

Homeopathy a system of medicine in which a patient is given minute doses of natural remedies that in larger quantities would produce symptoms of the disease itself

Hormone a chemical substance produced by the body that regulates or controls aspects such as growth and development

Immunosuppressant a drug that inhibits the body's immune system, used to prevent rejection of transplanted organs

Influenza a viral disease producing high temperature, sore throat, runny nose, headache, dry cough and muscle pain

Insulin a hormone that regulates the level of glucose in the blood

Leukemia a type of cancer in which white blood cells replace normal blood, causing infection, anemia, bleeding and other disorders

Lobotomy an operation in which nerves to the prefrontal lobe of the brain are severed

Malaria an infectious disease caused by a parasite that is transmitted by the bite of infected mosquitoes

Marburg virus a severe viral infection causing high fever, hemorrhaging, rashes, vomiting and often death

Meningitis a viral or bacterial infection of the meninges (membranes that protect the brain and spinal cord), causing severe headaches, vomiting, fever and sometimes death

Naturopathy a system of medicine based on the belief that diet, mental state, exercise, breathing and other natural factors are central to the cause and treatment of disease

Obesity a condition in which a person's weight is more than 20% higher than is recommended for that person's height

Ovulation the ripening and discharge of eggs from a woman's ovary for possible fertilization

Parkinson's disease a disease of the nervous system that causes tremors and lack of co-ordination in the limbs

Pellagra a disease caused by a deficiency of niacin

PET scanner a positron emission tomography scanner that produces an image of a cross-section of part of the body, usually the brain, showing the chemical interactions taking place

Polio short for poliomyelitis, a severe, infectious viral disease affecting young people. It inflames the brainstem and spinal cord, sometimes leading to paralysis

Retrovirus a virus whose genetic information is contained in RNA, not DNA. RNA stands for ribonucleic acid. The RNA molecule is found in all living cells and is essential for the manufacture of proteins according to the instructions carried by genes

Rickets a disease caused by a deficiency in vitamin D that causes the bones to become soft

SARS abbreviation of severe acute respiratory syndrome: a viral disease related to pneumonia that originated in China in 2002, causing fever, breathing difficulties and sometimes death

Scarlet fever an infectious disease common in childhood

Schizophrenia a mental disease marked by a breakdown in the connection between thoughts, feelings and actions, and frequently accompanied by false beliefs

Scurvy a disease caused by a lack of vitamin C

Septicaemia a disease caused by poisonous micro-organisms in the bloodstream

Smallpox a highly contagious disease caused by the poxvirus and marked by high fever and the formation of pustules on the skin

Sulphonamides a range of drugs used to treat bacterial infections before the development of antibiotics in the 1940s

Syphilis a serious sexually transmitted disease that effects many parts of the body including the genitals, brain, skin and nervous tissue

Tuberculosis an infectious disease that causes small swellings to form on mucous membranes. It usually effects the lungs

Ultrasound scanning a type of scan that uses high-frequency sound waves reflecting off internal body parts to create images, especially of the fetus in the womb

Vaccine a preparation that uses weakened or dead microbes of the kind that cause a particular disease, administered to stimulate the body's immune system to produce antibodies against that disease

Vitamin an organic substance that is essential in small quantities to nutrition

Yellow fever an infectious, often fatal viral disease of warm climates, transmitted by mosquitoes and marked by high fever, hemorrhaging, jaundice and vomiting of blood

Timeline

Breakthrough dates in the history of 20th century medicine

Events	Dates	People
	1900	**1900** Starling and Bayliss discover the first hormone
		1901 Karl Landsteiner classifies human blood groups
		1906 Frederick Hopkins discovers vitamins
1918-1919 Influenza epidemic kills around 25 million people	**1920**	
1921 Discovery of insulin		**1928** Alexander Fleming discovers Penicillin
	1940	
1944 Penicillin comes into widespread use	**1950**	
		1953 James Watson and Francis Crick identify structure of DNA
		Leroy Stevens discovers stem cells
		John Gibbon invents the heart-lung machine
		1954 Jonas Salk develops the first vaccine against polio
	1960	
		1967 Christiaan Barnard carries out the first successful heart transplant
	1970	
		1973 Godfrey Hounsfield invents the CAT scanner
1978 Smallpox is eradicated		
The first test-tube baby is born		
	1980	
1981 AIDS becomes a worldwide epidemic		
	1990	
1997 Avian flu spreads from birds to humans		

Further information

Books

A Social History of Medicines in the Twentieth Century: To be Taken Three Times a Day, John K. Crellin, Pharmaceutical Products Press, 2004

Aimed at older readers, this looks at the social and medical influences on the use of medicine in the twentieth century.

Blood and Guts: A Short History of Medicine, Roy W.W. Norton, 2003

Medicine in the Twentieth Century, Roger Cooter and John Pickstone (editors), Routledge, 2002

A series of essays, intended for older readers.

Milestones of Medicine: The Eventful 20th Century, Reader's Digest editors, Reader's Digest, 2001

Chronicles the medical breakthroughs of the century.

The Story of Medicine: From Acupuncture to X Rays, Judy Lindsay, Oxford University Press, 2003

The history of medicine from ancient to modern times, organized in thematic chapters.

Technology All Around Us: Medicine, Kristina Routh, Smart Apple Media, 2005

About the cutting-edge technologies used in medicine.

Invisible Enemies: Stories of Infectious Disease, Jeanette Farrell, Farrar, Straus & Giroux, 2005

Covers 7 infectious diseases from plague to AIDS.

Surgery: An Illustrated History, Ira M. Rutkow, Mosby-Year Book, 1993

Websites

www.bbc.co.uk/history/discovery/medicine
Articles on medical success stories, including the eradication of smallpox.

www.historylearningsite.co.uk/history_of_medicine.htm
A look at the important trends and people in the history of medicine, with the emphasis on modern medicine.

http://profiles.nlm.nih.gov/
Biographies of important figures in the development of modern medicine.

www.channel4.com/history/microsites/H/history/browse/medical.html
A series of on-line essays, including ones on thalidomide and the 1918-19 flu pandemic.

www.who.int/en/
The website for the World Health Organization.

Read all about the work they are doing to help alleviate diseases around the world.

www.cwru.edu/artsci/dittrick/site2/
Dittrick Medical History Center site with exhibits and a link to an excellent list of medical museums, archives and libraries in the USA.

www.si.edu/science_and_technology/health_and_human_sciences
The Smithsonian's health and human science website with information on brain research, molecules, anatomy, polio and more.

www.schoolscience.co.uk/content/4/biology/abpi/history/history11.html
Pages 11-16 of this link of the site address medicine from 1900-2000, covering such topics as infectious diseases, diabetes and insulin, genetics, the human genome, technology, and more.

www.nlm.nih.gov/hmd/index.html
Gateway to the United States National Library of Medicine. Educational links, links to current and upcoming exhibitions, as well as nearly 60,000 images in a variety of media illustrating the social and historically specific aspects of medicine.

Places to visit

Museum of Science, Boston, MA
www.mos.org
On the cutting edge of science education, innovative, interactive exhibits range from bugs and supernovas to the medical x-ray and contemporary medical imaging techniques.

National Museum of Health and Medicine, Washington, D.C.
http://nmhm.washingtondc.musum
More than 350 collections document the practice of medicine from the Civil War to the present.

John P. McGovern Museum of Health & Medical Science, Houston, TX
www.mhms.org
A unique health and science education facility housing the Jim Hickox Amazing Body Pavilion, a larger than life walking tour through the human body. Also mounts exhibitions that focus on topics such as nanobiotechnology.

Science Museum of Minnesota, St. Paul, MN
www.smm.org
Perhaps the most popular museum in the Upper Midwest, SMM presents exhibitions on the history of science, medicine and technology.